Telemicrosurgery

Philippe A. Liverneaux • Stacey H. Berner
Michael S. Bednar • Sijo J. Parekattil
Gustavo Mantovani Ruggiero
Jesse C. Selber
Editors

Telemicrosurgery

Robot Assisted Microsurgery

Springer

Editors
Philippe A. Liverneaux
Centre de Chirurgie Orthopédique
et de la Main (CCOM)
Hôpitaux Universitaires de Strasbourg
Unité SOS Main
Illkirch CX
France

Stacey H. Berner
Department of Orthopedic Surgery
Northwest Hospital
Baltimore, MD
USA

Michael S. Bednar
Chicago Orthopaedic Surgery
and Rehabilitation
Loyola University
Maywood, IL
USA

Sijo J. Parekattil
Robotic Surgery and Urology
Winter Haven Hospital &
University of Florida
Winter Haven, FL
USA

Gustavo Mantovani Ruggiero
São Paolo Hand Center
Sao Paolo
Brazil

Jesse C. Selber
Department of Plastic Surgery
M.D. Anderson Cancer Center
Houston, TX
USA

ISBN 978-2-8178-0390-6 ISBN 978-2-8178-0391-3 (eBook)
DOI 10.1007/978-2-8178-0391-3
Springer Paris Heidelberg New York Dordrecht London

Library of Congress Control Number: 2012953556

Printed on acid-free paper

Springer is part of Springer Science+Business Media (www.springer.com)

Foreword

Robotic assisted surgery may conjure images of science fiction; however, it has become a modern reality. Some traditionalists within the medical community have expressed skepticism about this approach, questioning the cost of this technology. However, it is difficult to ignore the fact that robotic assisted surgery has extraordinary potential. Some of our colleagues are testing the outer limits of microsurgery with preliminary work on suturing capillary vessels. We may question the benefits of applying this technology. Is our primary purpose the achievement of a surgical prowess? Perhaps the cynic may draw this conclusion, but in fact we have likely only begun to tap into the vast potential of this emerging discipline. When Pasteur enlightened about the existence of microbes, and the necessity for strict hygiene and sterile technique, a famous English surgeon uttered the short-sighted sentence: "Anyway, microbes, I do not see them, and if they exist I cut them in half with my knife!"

So as we evaluate dramatically new technological advances, let us not forget that many concepts and devices that we would now consider indispensible to modern medicine likely were not initially embraced. Amongst the tremendous enhancements that robotics has enabled are:

- Improved comfort and ergonomics of our workstation
- Increasing safety in sterilization of the operative field
- Creation of a three dimensional "augmented reality"
- Ultra-precise instrument control through the de-multiplication effect, resulting in improvement of our surgical procedures

In this book you will discover many facets of ultra-modern robotic assisted surgery. Philippe Liverneaux has pioneered many of these techniques. Along with his colleagues and co-authors from the RAMSES society, he provides world class educational experiences at the magnificent Ircad training facility in Strasbourg, France. The mission of these training courses, the RAMSES society and this text are to raise awareness of the expanded applications of Robotic Surgery. This will help move this technology to its rightful place at the forefront amongst surgical advances and hopefully will add a great tool to our daily practices.

Paris, France   Christophe L. Mathoulin M.D

Preface

Participating in February 2007 at an EWAS lecture (European Wrist Arthroscopy Society) organized by Christophe Mathoulin, I was given the opportunity to take a tour of IRCAD-EITS in Strasbourg (Institut de Recherche sur les Cancers de l'Appareil Digestif – European Institute for Tele-Surgery).Taking a peek through an open door at the back of the conference room, I was pretty much awed to find myself looking at some sort of giant metallic spider, no different from those in horror movies, attempting to swallow a little pig fast asleep. I was told the beast's name was "Zeus", and that it was a remote controlled surgical robot for surgeons to practice laparoscopy. It happened Zeus was as a matter-of-fact the ancestor of the DaVinci® robot. It had already been used in 2001 by Jacques Marescaux during an outstanding surgical performance, a transatlantic cholecystectomy, transatlantic because the surgeon operated in New York a patient anesthetized in Strasbourg, separated by more than 5,000 km [1]. I was furthermore allowed to experience Zeus for a little while, far much time than necessary for me to succumb to the robot's swiftness and docility.

From this day on, I decided I would not rest until I could adapt such a robot to the surgical discipline I performed daily for so many years: microsurgery. Why should robotics be solely reserved to general surgeons? I spoke to Didier Mutter, Jacques Marescaux's assistant, who introduced me to David Douglas, technical engineer at Intuitive Surgical™, the company which builds and sells DaVinci® robots, precisely at the time when the latter tended to replace obsolescent Zeus robots. David told me IRCAD-EITS was a training center in robotics, training surgeons worldwide in order to help them master the DaVinci® robot. I was invited by David to such a training session, provided I committed myself to developing innovative surgical techniques using the robot. I had no other restriction than to be creative!!! I needn't be told this twice… I quickly had the opportunity to work at the task in May 2007 when Chihab Taleb, a resident in Strasbourg, asked for a thesis for the Microsurgery Diploma. I proposed that his work focused on a neologism, *telemicrosurgery*, so as to transpose the telesurgical concept to microsurgery. Eric Nectoux, another resident coming from Lille and at the time spending 6 months in Strasbourg, offered his help to develop this new technical concept. This is how telemicrosurgery, alias robotics applied to microsurgery, all begun…

The first studies focused on the rat, then pigs and eventually human cadavers. While Chihab focused on vascular anastomosis, Eric worked on nervous sutures

[2, 3], both studies leading to major papers as first authors. During 6 months, week after week, we worked for hours attempting to define the best way to perform surgical repair of many different histological tissues: arteries, nerves, veins, tendons, muscles, ligaments, skin, etc. We learned step by step progressively how to install the robot, display its arms, and master the multiple pedals and handles. After a few months, we decided we were geared up to perform one of the most microsurgically challenging procedures: a macro-replantation of the limb. After a preliminary feasibility study in a pig cadaver, I bought a live pig from IRCAD-EITS and Brice Hérain, one of David Douglas' colleagues, booked an operating room between two DaVinci® training sessions. A go-getting surgical team was about to experience an outstanding March 31, 2008: Brice installed two robots, Dominique Lazner and Muriel Renard (our scrub nurses) managed the surgical field and all surgical needs, while three surgeons Chihab, Eric and I took turns on both surgical consoles. The procedure last 5 h including installation of the robots, amputation of the forelimb of the pig and its replantation [4].

We felt the need to share our experience by creating a scientific society, the RASH Society (Robotic-Assisted Surgery of the Hand/www.rash-society.org) and a bi-annual workshop at IRCAD-EITS promoting telemicrosurgical teaching on biological models (earthworms, chicken thighs, etc.). Participants came from Europe, South and North America with Mike Bednar (USA), Gustavo Mantovani (Brazil) and Stacey Berner (USA) as guest experts to coach the surgeons attending the workshops.

After having developed laboratory telemicrosurgery, a new step had to be taken forward: clinical practice. I first thought difficulties would arise from our using the robot for microsurgery, as in the USA the FDA (Food and Drug Administration) delivers authorizations for the robot to selected surgical disciplines with regard to selected surgical procedures! In France, there are no such restrictions, provided the robot is used for a surgical procedure, regardless of the surgery performed. As a matter of fact, logistical, practical and financial difficulties were eventually at stake. Financially speaking the University Hospitals of Strasbourg (HUS) had bought a DaVinci® robot a couple of years previously, and the surgical teams involved in using the robot had to resign to postpone for 2 years the acquisition of other biomedical equipments. I therefore had to comply myself to these financial decisions, and at this point my warmest thanks go to Michèle Brid, our operating room manager, for having managed to save 20,000€ in a year, allowing us to enter the very select club of surgical teams in Strasbourg licensed to use DaVinci®. Practically speaking, I then had to sign the charter clearly stipulating that there were no scrub nurses attributed to DaVinci®, my own surgical team being responsible for the surgical procedure when using the robot. My team is located 10 km from the hospital where the robot is located, and the robot could not be moved away easily. It suddenly became evident that difficulties would arise, since my surgical team would have to operate in an "unknown" hospital, in an "unknown" surgical ward, with all new surgical equipment. Nothing stopped us. Muriel and Dominique were always by my side when the mood was down. Surgical procedures were performed at a steady rhythm of 1 per month, while thinking of new vascular or nervous indications with Sybille Facca and Stéphanie Gouzou. Time passing by, along with our increasing experience, it seems peripheral nerve microsurgery is the best indication for telemicrosurgery. The first case of peripheral nerve surgery was performed by Stacey Berner in the USA. For legal reasons, authorizations for this procedure with a DaVinci® robot were given provided I assisted him as a hotline. Unfortunately, video transmission between Baltimore and Strasbourg was unavailable, and we managed to perform this ulnar nerve graft together thanks to Skype™! However the robot was no bonus compared to a conventional microscope, since this telemicrosurgery was performed through an open approach.

Thus, it was urgent to redefine new openings for telemicrosurgery; the concept of minimally-invasive soft tissue surgery of the limbs became evident. Using a robot for telemicrosurgery isn't *per se* of great interest, since the same procedure can be performed by conventional microsurgery. We went back to IRCAD-EITS labs to study the feasibility of minimally-invasive telemicrosurgery. The forearm, and more precisely the median nerve, was our surgical experimental paradigm. The number and width of surgical approaches needed to be defined, along with both the possibility to create a surgical cavity where all surgical instruments would rejoin and the topographic maintenance of such a cavity during all the procedure. These solutions are still under development, with help of Kiyohito Naito (Japan) and Thierry Lequint (Belgium), both very actively concerned by minimally invasive approaches. Some time later we developed a minimally-invasive technique for brachial plexus surgery using carbon dioxide insufflation with Gustavo Mantovani (Brazil) and Catherine Mohr (USA) from the labs at Intuitive Surgical™, Sunnyvale, CA.

Since we already had a reasonable experience of surgical repair of brachial plexus with Frédéric Lebailly and Sybille Facca, we performed the minimally-invasive technique developed at Sunnyvale in our first cases. The first case was a brachial plexus biopsy for a nervous tumor, and the second case was the removal of a recurrence of a 5 cm long desmoid tumor of the brachial plexus by an approach less than a centimetre long. Minimally-invasive telemicrosurgery was born!

It was in Sunnyvale, at the Intuitive Surgical™ headquarters, that all six founders of the RAMSES (Robotic Assisted Micro-Surgery and Endoscopic Surgery/www.roboticmicrosurgeons.org) first met (that is Stacey Berner (USA), Mike Bednar (USA), Sijo Parekattil (USA), Jesse Selber (USA), Gustavo Mantovani (Brazil) and myself). It was Jesse who first thought of RAMSES, inside the white limo which was bringing us to the labs. Sijo organized the first congress of the RAMSES at Orlando in November 2011. What will be the next step?

This book takes stock of telemicrosurgery since its birth until now. History of both microsurgery and telesurgery is told by pioneers in these domains, Yoshikazu Ikuta and Jacques Marescaux. Telemicrosurgery goes upriver to the source of both disciplines. Firstly surgical robots and their functioning are precisely described by renowned experts who master this technology. Secondly training is seriously framed by precise pedagogic protocols and well standardized models. Authors who define telemicrosurgery do not leave any room for improvisation. Thirdly come all experimental models proposed by founder members of the RAMSES. At last, the most complete description of clinical applications is given by means of several transversal surgical disciplines: peripheral nerve surgery, skin/muscle flap surgery, plastic surgery and urology. It is Catherine Mohr, woman whose scientific culture is as vast as a university library, along with an acute practical sense, which will give us hints as for the future of surgical robots. Special thanks go to Christophe Mathoulin and Terry Whipple, famous names in arthroscopy, who provided by their insight a parallel between their accomplished discipline and the rising telemicrosurgery.

Strasbourg, France Philippe André Liverneaux, M.D., Ph.D

References

1. Marescaux J, Leroy J, Gagner M et al (2001) Transatlantic robot-assisted telesurgery. Nature 413:379–380
2. Nectoux E, Taleb C, Liverneaux P (2009) Nerve repair in telemicrosurgery: an experimental study. J Reconstruc Microsurg 25:261–265
3. Taleb C, Nectoux E, Liverneaux P (2008) Telemicrosurgery: a feasability study in a rat model. Chir Main 28:104–108
4. Taleb C, Nectoux E, Liverneaux P (2009) Limb replantation with two robots: a feasibility study in a pig model. Microsurg 29:232–235

Contents

Part I

General

History of Microsurgery

1

Yoshikazu Ikuta

1.1 Introduction

As microsurgery is a confluence of the microscope and vascular surgery, one can understand the history of microsurgery through an overview of these two histories.

When we look back on the history of the microscope, there are four generations. That is, the first generation is about 330 years from the development of the physical microscope in 1590 to its application to surgery in 1921. The second takes place over the 40 years from 1921 to the year of first report of microscopic vascular surgery by Jacobson in 1960 [51]. And the third is over the 40 years from 1960 to the development of high magnification microscope by Kuroshima in 2004 [63]. The fourth and final period is the one from 2000 to the present. After the application of microscope to the field of surgery, I would like to designate these as Classic Binocular Dissection Surgery Period (1921–1960), Standard Microsurgery Period (1960–2000), and Fine Microsurgery Period (2000–2011).

1.2 History of the Microscope and Its Application to the Surgery

Although there are some conflicts as to whether the first developer of the microscope was Janssen (Holland, 1590), Drebbel (Holland, 1621), or Fontana (Italy, 1618), it is true that it was developed between the sixteenth and seventeenth centuries in Europe.

Blood circulation theory by Harvey (1628) cited in [72, 73] and "Micrographia" by Hooke [42] and so on was the first generation works which are described accord-

Y. Ikuta, M.D.
Hiroshima University School of Medicine,
Hand and Microsurgery Center,
Nakashima Bldg 2F4-11, Nakajima-cho, Naka-ku, Hiroshima 730-0811, Japan
e-mail: blueskyikuta@gmail.com

P. Liverneaux et al. (eds.), *Telemicrosurgery*,
DOI 10.1007/978-2-8178-0391-3_1, © Springer-Verlag France 2013

ing to scientific observation using the microscope, and these publications left a strong impression on people as to the usefulness of the microscope and the development of the new scientific world. In 1673, Leeuwenhoek published "Philosophical transaction," which is the first book of scientific observation of microorganisms, and that this kind of work should not be done without the use of the microscope.

The microscope was used as a tool of surgery by Holmgren [41], in 1923. He resected a promontory using 10 diopter of binocular dissecting microscope [41]. After that, many surgeons used a microscope, such as Perritt [87] and Barraquer [4] in the field of ophthalmology; Jacobson et al. [51] in the field of vascular surgery; Ito et al. [49], Smith [96], Michon et al. [77] in the field of peripheral nerve; Kurze [65], Jacobson and Donaghy [50], Malis [69], Donaghy and Yasargil [29], Walz [111], and Swolin [101] in the field of neurosurgery; David et al. [25] in the field of gynecology.

The microscope has been improved by introduction of a coaxial illumination system (Littman 1954 cited in [45]), a ceiling suspension system [4], and a motorized zoom objective lens [108].

Since 1970, in the field of orthopedic and plastic and reconstructive surgery, as replantation surgery and vascularized free tissue transplantation spread all over the world as standard surgery, the microscope for the surgeon has become common place, and improvements in the microscope has adapted to the request of surgeon. For example, illumination is brighter, focus and zoom can be controlled with a foot pedal or audio response unit, and operator and assistant are able to see the same operative field and video and still photo functions are routine. I would like to introduce some modern microscopes which are used in the operation theater. There are OPMI series by Carl-Zeiss Co. Ltd., M525/MS3 series by Leica Co. Ltd., and OME series by Olympus Co. Ltd. and some excellent idea of supporting post, such as "robotic stand" by Leica, "counterbalanced arm" by Olympus, and "overhead stand" by Mitaka Co. Ltd., complete coaxial illumination system, electric-powered operative field moving system, and so on. The most distinguished development in microscope technology is the high magnification microscope MW50/YOH series by Mitaka Co. Ltd., which has 50× magnification with a 200-mm working distance. With the appearance of this kind of microscope, the new world of so-called "ultra-microsurgery" [47], "super-microsurgery" [114], or "half-millimeter microsurgery" [64] can be developed [64].

1.3 History of Vascular Surgery

The first paper of vascular surgery is "A new technique of treating an aneurysm" in Medical Observations and Inquiries by Lambert in 1761 [67]. According to this literature, on June 15, 1759, Hallowell treated an injured brachial artery by means suture repair rather than ligation [35]. After that, there are many reports of treatment of large size vessel such as femoral artery (Travers 1816 cited in [45]), carotid artery (Czerny 1881 cited in [45]), portal [32], and vein at the inguinal region (Schede in 1882 cited in [45], Keen in 1900 cited in [45]).

With regard to end-to-end anastomosis of vessels Jassinowski [52], described needle, suture material, and instruments for animal experiments at first, and Murphy [80] described anastomosis of human vessels.

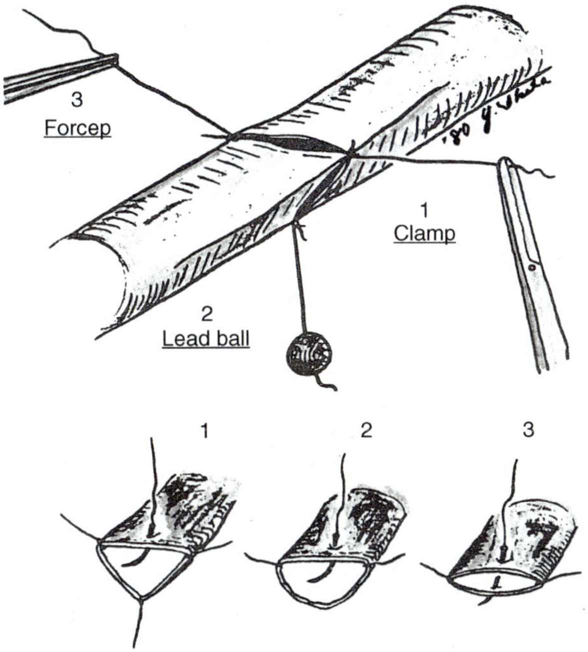

Fig. 1.1 Three-stay suture method after Carrel [15] and asymmetric biangulation two-stay sutures method

These days, the most distinguished achievement is a paper of “La technique opératoire des anastomoses vasculaires et la transplantation des viscères” by Carrel (Fig. 1.1) [15]. He described the famous three points stay suture method in this paper. In spite of more than one hundred years since the publication of this paper, it is neither stale nor old, but it is fundamental and passed on as asymmetric biangulation two-stay sutures method. After that, one might guess that a standard technique of vascular surgery should be almost established by some papers, such as *Blood Vessel Surgery and Its Application* [33], vascular treatment at the time of Balkan war (Weitung and Vollbrecht 1912–1913 cited in [45]), and report of treatment of peripheral arteries (Goodman 1914 cited in [45]). After many reports of a treatment method of large vessel, a method of angiography [88], an artery graft [66, 100], and artificial vessels are developed and utilized in clinical cases (Edwards 1955, Julian 1957 cited in [53, 102]).

1.4 History of Small Vessel Anastomosis

In 1960, Julius H. Jacobson and Ernesto L. Suarez reported “Microsurgery in anastomosis of small vessels” in *Surgical Forum*. This is the first paper of microscopic vascular anastomosis in the world. After that, there are many reports about efforts to achieve good results with small vessel anastomosis and its application to tissue grafts, such as in the description of tube and cuff ligature and its application to clinical cases [7, 93], and description of suture material [43], or microangiography technique [5].

In 1956, Androsov developed a suture device using a tantalum staple [2], Inokuchi developed a suture device using the 22A alloy staple in 1961 [48], and Sterling reported another device using a staple in 1959 [97] and 1960 [23]. Drawbacks of these mechanical suture devices are as follows: it is difficult to use it when both cut ends of the vessel are not long enough, and sometimes it is difficult to invert the vessel ends, especially in the case of arteriosclerosis.

On the other hand, in 1960, there are many important reports, such as fundamental studies of cyanoacrylate adhesive (Eastman 90, Aron-Alpha) by Nathan et al. [82] and Kessler and Carton [56] and ring-pin suture method by Nakayama et al. [81]. This ring-pin method is succeeded as UniLink 3M precise microvascular anastomotic device [85] [55] and GEM microvascular anastomosis system by WonderWorks Co. Ltd. We modified this ring with absorbable material (poly-L-lactic acid), and good result in experimental study, but it was not marketed (Ikuta et al. [47]). As the other reports, there are trials of patch graft to reduce constriction of suture site [24], development of tantalum ring [90], for limb and kidney transplantation using dog [68]. In 1961 and 1962, there are many reports of utilization of adhesive [39] and patch graft [26], and mechanical dilatation of vessel ends [40].

From this year to 1964, some new methods of end-to-end anastomosis are reported such as mechanical suture [23, 75, 97, 98] and temporary stent insertion into the vessel lumen and so on [3, 70, 79]. Fundamental research of suture materials or/and instruments [12, 16–18, 22, 91, 110, 113] and studies of adhesives [6, 30, 71] are reported. And Siegel et al. [94, 95] reported an application of an electric coagulation machine instead of manual suture. The most two interesting experiments in 1965 are digital amputation and replantation in the monkey, by Buncke and Schulz [14], and composite graft in the dog by Krizek et al. [62]. These studies represent the dawn of a new world of microvascular surgery. Miraculously, the first replantation of a completely severed thumb occurred in Japan by Komatsu and Tamai [61], in this same year. As the background contribution to these surgeries, there is another relevant field of study which is the application of microscopic technique in peripheral nerve. Ito in Japan reported the fascicular suture of peripheral nerve [49], based on the intraneural topographic atlas in 1976. His experimental work of peripheral nerve started in Hiroshima before 1962. At that time, I was a medical student, and he was our teacher. Smith [96] in New York also reported his special technique for repairing peripheral nerve, as fascicular matching [96]. Thereafter, Bora [8] and Hakstian [34] contributed to fascicular oriented repair of the nerves [8, 34]. In 1966, two memorable experimental studies are reported by Buncke, which is a replantation of a rabbit ear and toe-to-hand transfer in a rhesus monkey [13]. In the field of material and technique of microsurgery, there are some interesting papers such as anastomosis using staple by Khodadad et al. [57–60] and Brunius et al. [10], fundamental technique by other many surgeons.

I started my experimental study of microvascular surgery in 1966. At that time, instruments for microsurgery were not suitable because there were too big. I designed several instruments for very fine micro-instruments including a microvascular clamp. The prototype of this clamp was handmade by myself, and ordered to Mizuho Ikakogyo Co. Ltd., in Japan later (Fig. 1.2). I reported the results of

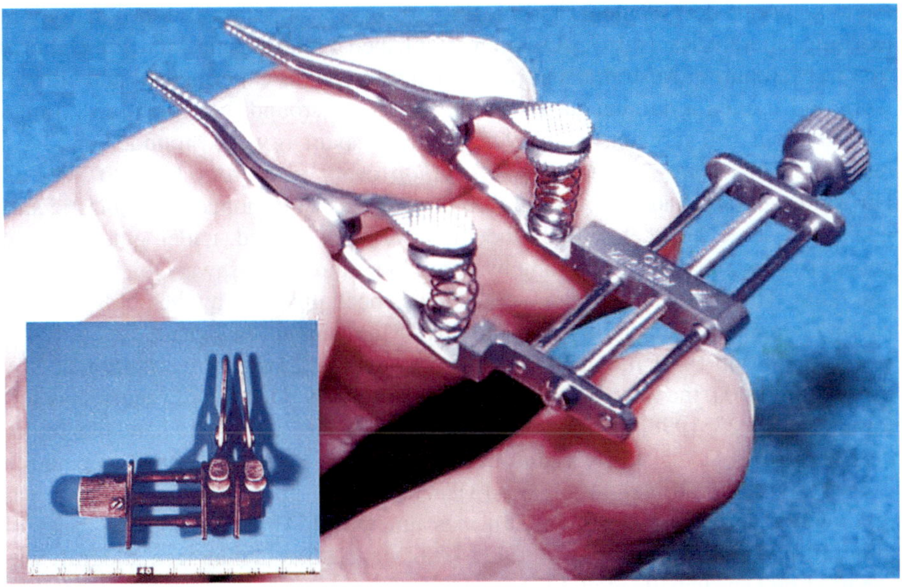

Fig. 1.2 Ikuta's prototype clamp designed in 1966 (*left small photo*) and modified to type L in 1968

anastomosis of artery and vein from 0.5 to 5 mm in diameter and some special instruments designed by myself (1968) [44]. My vascular clamp is even a little bit large and heavy, but because of this feature, it is easy to use under microscope.

From the middle of the 1960s to 1970s, diverse fields of clinical applications in microsurgery were developed. John Cobbett published a paper on the basic and standard technique of microvascular surgery in Surgical Clinics of North America in 1967 [20]. He stressed asymmetric biangulation stay sutures. Donaghy and Yasargil succeeded in a bypass operation for an embolism of the middle cerebral artery in 1967 [29], experimental skeletal muscle graft by Tamai et al. in 1968 [103], and second toe-to-hand transfer by Chen et al. in 1968 [19], and hallux-to-thumb was done by Cobbett in 1968 [21], also.

Entering the 1970s, like many flowers blooming at once, various experimental studies and clinical applications were reported; for example, transplantation of omentum to the denuded scalp created by the removal of a squamous cell carcinoma by McLean et al. [76], first case of free flap transfer in the world by Harii et al. [37], pectoralis major muscle transfer by Shanghai group (1973) [89], gracilis muscle transfer by Harii and Ohmori [36, 38], pectoralis major muscle transfer into forearm by Ikuta et al. [46], vascular nerve graft by Taylor (1976), and vascularized bone graft by Ueba and Fujikawa [109], Taylor et al. [105, 106], Buncke [11], Strauch et al. [99], Tamai et al. [104], McCullough et al. [74], Oestrup et al. [84], and Doi et al. [28] were reported. In the field of peripheral nerve microsurgery, experimental and clinical developments are achieved by Samii and Wallenburg [92], Terzis et al. [107], Williams and Terzis [112], Millesi et al. [78], and Brunelli [9]. In addition to the tremendous development of clinical microsurgery, there was a lot of activity in teaching laboratories. In 1972, O'Brien established a microsurgical teaching laboratory in Melbourne, Australia, and performed tremendous experimental and clinical work and trained a number of microsurgeons from around the world [83]. Tamai trained about 150 surgeons from 1972 in Nara, Japan, as well. I founded and have held *The Hiroshima Microsurgery Workshop* every year from 1976 to 2001 in Hiroshima, Japan, and more than 1,300 participants of orthopedic and plastic surgeon, and some medical school students have been trained, under guidance and person to person technical teaching by Kino, Yoshimura, Fujisawa, Doi, Miyamoto, and Ikuta. This personal training workshop has been inherited by the public organization of Japanese Society of Reconstructive Microsurgery in Japan.

From 1980 to 1990, innumerable autogenous tissue grafts were reported, and by the end of 1990s, the new period commenced. In 1999, Dubernard reported as follows, On Sept 23, 1998, we transplanted the right distal forearm and hand of a brain-dead man, aged 41 years on to a man aged 48 years who had had traumatic amputation of the distal third of his right forearm [31]. And follow-up data of this first case was reported by Kanitakis that the result was unhappy [54]. Some another cases of allograft of human hand are reported [84, 86]. In 2006, a human face allograft was reported by Devauchelle et al. [27].

These allograft of human hand or face is the meaning of opening another new world of microsurgery, but we have to consider that these clinical successful cases are supported by immunosuppressive agent, and we have to consider a comment by the American Society for Surgery of the Hand in 1998 as follows: "The risk-to-benefit ratio for the transplantation of a cadaveric hand/forearm has yet to be convincingly established. Until current immunosuppressive pharmacology has vastly improved, hand and forearm transplantation should be considered a high-risk procedure that is still in a very experimental phase."

Conclusion

At the closing of this chapter, I would like to mention the limitation of microsurgery. Up to 2000, the mainstream of microsurgery is as follows. Under the microscope and 20–30 magnification, using 10-0 or 11-0 monofilament nylon suture, vessels in diameter from 3.0 to 0.5 mm are treated. In 1979, Acland stated that the limitation of minimum diameter of vessel is 0.3 mm in diameter [1]. Looming factors against proceeding with more fine microsurgery are low-magnifying optic aid, large suture material, and tremor and awkward movement of the human hand. To solve these problems, surgeons strive to develop mechanical suture devices, fine suture material and needles, high-magnifying microscopes, and robot or manipulator systems.

In the beginning of 1980, I utilized two manipulators to treat cells which were made by Nagashima Co. Ltd. to perform microvascular anastomoses (Fig. 1.3) and a stereoscopic microscope (DXC-1850 by Sony) using electric controlled polarized goggles (Fig. 1.4). The successful ratio of arterial anastomoses ranged from 0.25 to 0.35 mm in diameter using 10-0, 11-0, and 12-0 nylon thread is 26 % (5 cases out of 19 arteries) [47]. The stereoscopic microscope is used as a high-magnification optic aid, at this time. In future, this tool

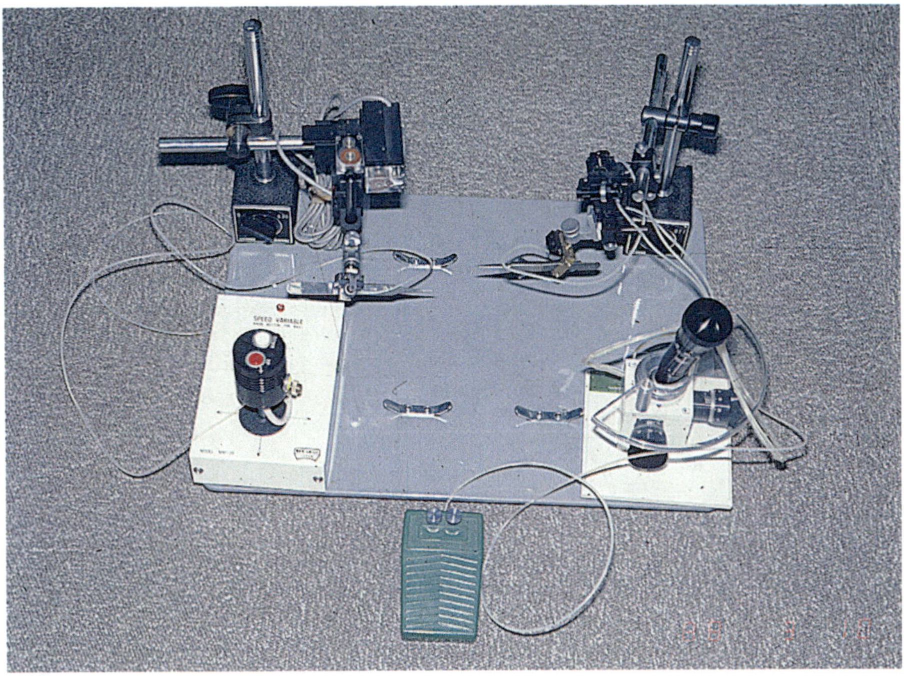

Fig. 1.3 Micromanipulator distributed from Nagashima Co. Ltd

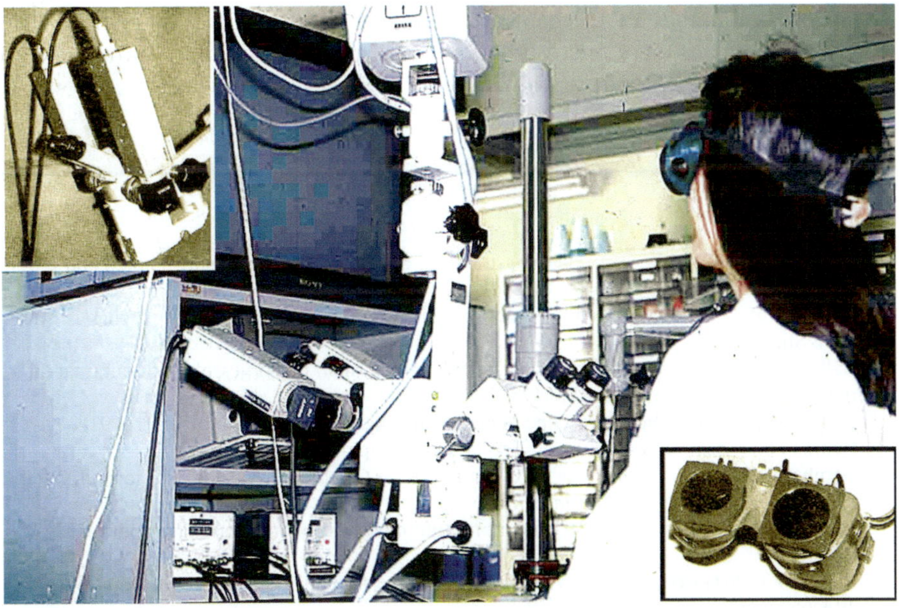

Fig. 1.4 Operator watching a monitor using a goggle. Two video camera heads attached to a microscope (*left upper*), and electric controlled polarized goggle (*right bottom*) is used to observe a monitor

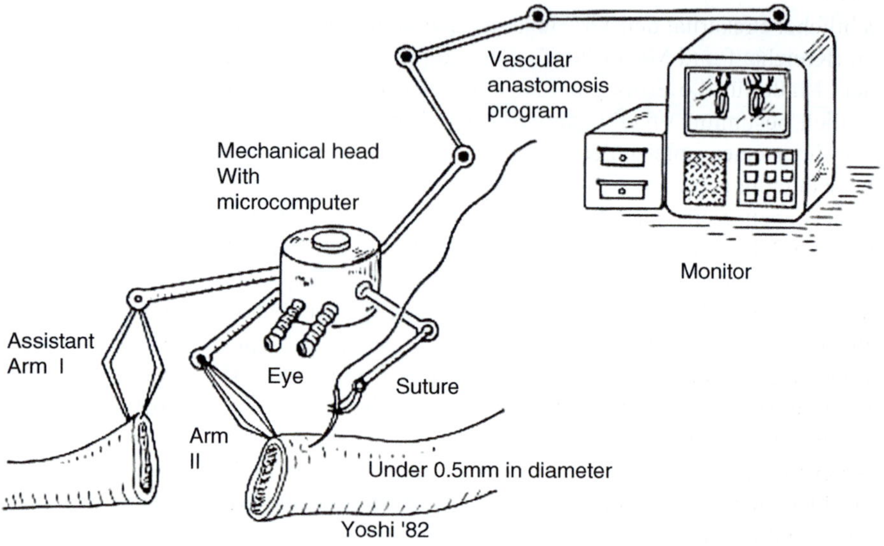

Fig. 1.5 The idea of intelligent robot system for microvascular anastomosis designed in 1983 [4]

is more meaningful because I am confident it can be used as a navigation system for a robot (Fig. 1.5).

In twenty-first century, we achieved high-magnification optic aid and the modern technology of mechanical movement systems with a computer brain. This new dimension of microsurgery is open in front of us, and we would like to take the first step into this new world.

References

1. Acland RD (1974) Microvascular anastomosis: a device for holding stay sutures and a new vascular clamp. Surgery 75:185–187
2. Androsov PI (1956) Blood supply of mobilized intestine used for an artificial esophagus. AMA Arch Surg 73:917–926
3. Ballinger WF, Fineberg C, Figlio D (1963) Repair of small blood vessels with minimal interruption of flow. J Surg Res 3:475–478
4. Barraquer JI (1956) The microscope in ocular surgery. Am J Ophthalmol 42:916–918
5. Bellman S (1953) Microangiography. Acta Radiol Suppl 102:1–104
6. Bernhard WF, Cummin AS, Vawter GF et al (1962) Closure of vascular incisions utilizing a new fixable adhesive. Surg Forum 13:231–233
7. Blakemore AH, Load JW Jr (1945) A nonsuture method of blood vessel anastomosis. JAMA 127:685
8. Bora FW (1967) Peripheral nerve repair in cats: the fascicular stitch. J Bone Joint Surg Am 49A:659–666
9. Brunelli G (1979) Long term results of nerve sutures and grafts. Microsurgery 1:27–31
10. Brunius U, Helander GL, Rudenstam CM et al (1966) Experience with staplers in anastomosing small blood vessels in dogs. Acta Chir Scand 131:30–37

11. Buncke HJ (1979) Microsurgical composite tissue trans-plantation. CV Mosby, St. Louis, pp 391–397
12. Buncke HJ Jr, Blackfield HM (1963) The vasoplegic effects of chlorpromazine. Plast Reconstr Surg 31:353–362
13. Buncke HJ, Buncke CM, Schulz WP (1966) Immediate Nicoladoni procedure in the Rhesus monkey for hallux to thumb transplantation utilizing microminiature anastomoses. Br J Surg 19:332–337
14. Buncke HJ, Schulz WP (1965) Experimental digital amputation and replantation. Plast Reconstr Surg 36:62–70
15. Carrel A (1902) La technique des anastomoses vasculaires et la transplantation des viscères. Lyon Med 98:859–864
16. Chase MD, Schwartz SI (1962) Consistent patency of 1.5 mm. Arterial anastomoses. Surg Forum 13:220–222
17. Chase MD, Schwartz SI (1963) Suture anastomosis of small arteries. Surg Gynecol Obstet 117:44–46
18. Chase MD, Schwartz SI, Rob C (1963) A technique of small artery anastomosis. Surg Gynecol Obstet 117:381–384
19. Chen ZW, Yang DY, Chang DS (1982) Microsurgery. Springer, Berlin, Heidelberg, New York, p 143
20. Cobbett JR (1967) Microvascular surgery. Surg Clin North Am 47:521–542
21. Cobbett JR (1969) Free digital transfer. J Bone Joint Surg 51B:677–679
22. Collins RE, Douglass FM (1964) Small vein anastomosis with and without operative microscope: a comparative study. AMA Arch Surg 88:740–742
23. Cooper P, Christie SG (1962) Development of the surgical stapler with emphasis on vascular anastomosis. Trans N Y Acad Sci 25:365–377
24. Crawford ES, Beal AC, Ellis PR Jr et al (1959) A technique permitting operation upon small arteries. Surg Forum 10:671–675
25. David A, Brackett RD, Garcia CR (1969) Effects of microsurgical removal of the rabbit uterotubal junction. Fertil Steril 20:250–257
26. De Leon AR, Crane PS et al (1961) Use of an autogenous vein patch in the performance of end-to-end anastomoses in small arteries. Surg Forum 12:258–259
27. Devauchelle B et al (2006) First human face allograft: early report. Lancet 368:203–209
28. Doi K, Tominaga S, Shibata T (1977) Bone grafts with microvascular anastomoses of vascular pedicles. J Bone Joint Surg Am 59A:809–815
29. Donaghy RMP, Yasargil MG (1967) Microvascular surgery. Georg Thiem/CV Mosby, Stuttgart/St. Louis, pp 87–125
30. Douglas B, Foster JH (1963) Union of severed arterial trunks and canalization without suture or prosthesis. Ann Surg 157:944
31. Dubernard JM et al (1999) Human hand allograft: report on first 6 months. Lancet 353:1315–1320
32. Eck NV (1877) Voprosno perevayazkie vorotuois voi. Predvaritelnoye sobstitjenye. Voen Med St Petersburg 130:1–2
33. Guthrie CC (1912) Blood vessel surgery and its applications. Longmans Green, New York, 16
34. Hakstian RW (1968) Funicular orientation by direct stimulation: an aid to peripheral nerve repair. J Bone Joint Surg 50A:1178–1186
35. Hallowell (1759) Cited by Eastcott HHG (1969) Arterial surgery. JB Lippincott, Philadelphia, p 235
36. Harii K (1979) Microvascular surgery in plastic surgery: free tissue transfer. J Microsurg 1:223–230
37. Harii K, Ohmori K, Ohmori S (1974) Hair transplantation with free scalp flap. Plast Reconstr Surg 53:259–270
38. Harii K, Ohmori K, Torii S (1976) Free gracilis muscle transplantation, with microneurovascular anastomoses for the treatment of facial paralysis. Plast Reconstr Surg 57:133–143
39. Healey JE Jr, Clerk RL et al (1962) Nonsuture repair of blood vessels. Ann Surg 155: 817–825

40. Hedberg SE (1962) Suture anastomosis of small vessels following relief of spasm by hydrostatic pressure dilatation. Ann Surg 155:51–59
41. Holmgren G (1923) Some experiences in surgery of otosclerosis. Acta Otolaryngol 5:460–466
42. Hooke R (1665) Micrographia. Manufactured in the United States of America. Dover Publications, Inc., New York
43. Hurwitt ES (1953) Intra-abdominal arterial anastomosis. An experimental study. Surgery 34:1043
44. Ikuta Y (1968) Studies on small vessel anastomosis. Hiroshima J Med Sci 17:285–311
45. Ikuta Y (1977) Microsurgery (In Japanese). Nankodo Co. Ltd., Tokyo, pp 7–14
46. Ikuta Y, Kubo T, Tsuge K (1976) Free muscle transplantation by microsurgical technique to treat severe Volkmann's contracture. Plast Reconstr Surg 58:407–411
47. Ikuta Y et al (1983) Challenge to limitations of microsurgery. Plastic Surg 26:620–625
48. Inokuchi K (1961) Stapling device for end-to-side anastomosis of blood vessels. Arch Surg 82:337–341
49. Ito J, Hirotani H, Yamamoto K (1976) Peripheral nerve repairs by the funicular suture technique. Acta Orthop Scand 47:283–289
50. Jacobson JH, Donaghy RMP (1962) Microsurgery as an aid to middle cerebral artery endarterectomy. J Neurosurg 19:108–115
51. Jacobson JH, Suarez EL (1960) Microsurgery in anastomosis of small vessels. Surg Forum 11:243–245
52. Jassinowski A (1889) Die Arterienaht: Eine experimentelle Studie. Inaug Diss Dorpat pp 1–103
53. Johnson RW (1967) Disease and medicine. B.T. Batsford Ltd., London
54. Kanitakis J et al (2003) Clinicopathologic features of graft rejection of the first human hand allograft. Transplant 76:688–693
55. Kawagoe H, Ikuta Y et al (1993) Analysis of vascular anastomosis with 3-M precise microvascular anastomosis system. J Microsug 6:197–202
56. Kessler LA, Carton CA (1960) Experimental studies in surgery of small blood vessels with the use of plastic adhesive. Prevention of aneurysmal dilatation. Surg Forum 11:403–404
57. Khodadad G (1969) Microvascular surgery. Microneurosurgery. The CV Mosby Company, St. Louis, pp 170–182, Chapter 13
58. Khodadad G, Lougheed WM (1964) Repair of small arteries with contact cement and Teflon graft. J Neurosurg 21:552–560
59. Khodadad G, Lougheed WM (1966) Repair and replacement of small arteries, microsuture technique. J Neurosurg 24:61–69
60. Khodadad G, Lougheed WM (1966) Stapling technique in segmental vein autografts and end-to-end anastomosis of small vein in dogs. Utilization of the operating microscope. J Neurosurg 24:855–864
61. Komatsu S, Tamai S (1968) Successful replantation of a completely cut-off thumb. Plast Reconstr Surg 42:374–377
62. Krizek TJ, Tani T, Desperez QQ et al (1965) Experimental transplantation of composite grafts by microvascular anastomosis. Plast Reconstr Surg 36:538–546
63. Kuroshima N (2004) Operative microscope with the most high magnification in the world and development of the most fine needle fitted with suture in the world(Japanese). Jap Reconstr Surg 17:159–160
64. Kuroshima N (2008) Modern technology-assisted microsurgery for innominate vessels. J Jap Soc Reconstr Microsug 21:347–352
65. Kurze T (1969) Extradural intracranial (middle fossa) approach to the internal auditory canal. J Neurosurg 19:1033–1037
66. Lam CR (1951) Resection of the descending thoracic aorta for aneurysm. Ann Surg 134:743–752
67. Lambert R (1761) A new method of treating an aneurysm. Medical observations and inquiries. William Johnston, London
68. Lapchinsky A (1960) Recent results of experimental transplantation of preserved limbs and kidneys and possible use of this technique in clinical practice. Ann N Y Acad Sci 87:539–571

69. Malis LI (1967) Bipolar coagulator in microsurgery. In: Donaghy RMP, Yasargil MG (eds) Microvascular surgery. Georg Thiem, Stuttgart, pp 126–130
70. Man B, Kohn Z (1962) Experiments on the anastomosis of small vessels. J Cardiovasc Surg 3: 195–200
71. Manax WG, Longerbeni J et al (1963) Plastic adhesive as an adjunct in suture anastomoses of small blood vessels. Surgery 54:663–666
72. Margotta R (1972) Medicina nei secoli (Translated in Japanese). Kodansha, Tokyo, pp 200–203, 211–213
73. Marti-Ibanes F (ed) (1962) The epic of medicine. Clarkson N. Ptter Inc., New York, pp 181–183
74. McCullough DW, Fredrickson JM (1973) Neurovascularized rib grafts to reconstruct mandibular defects. Can J Otolaryngol 2:96–100
75. McDonald JC, Fukuda A (1966) Rabbit renal homografts. Technique for grafts to the neck. Surgery 59:1156
76. McLean DH, Buncke HJ (1972) Autotransplant of omentum to large scalp defect with microsurgical revascularization. Plast Reconstr Surg 49:268–273
77. Michon J (1975) Nerve suture today traumatic nerve Lesions of the Upper Limb. Churchill Livingstone, Edinburgh, pp 69–74
78. Millesi H, Meissl G, Berger A (1976) Further experience with interfascicular grafting of the median, ulnar, and radial nerve. J Bone Joint Surg 58A:209–218
79. Mozes M, Man B, Agmon M et al (1963) Small vessel anastomosis. Surgery 54:609–611
80. Murphy JB (1897) Resection of arteries and veins injured in continuity end-to-end suture: experimental and clinical research. Med Rec 51:73
81. Nakayama K, Tamiya T, Yamamoto K et al (1962) A simple new apparatus for small vessel anastomosis (free autograft of the sigmoid included). Surgery 52:918–931
82. Nathan HS, Nachlas MM, Solomon RD (1960) Nonsuture closure of arterial incisions using a rapidly-polymerizing adhesive. Ann Surg 152:648–659
83. O'Brien BM (1977) Microvascular reconstructive surgery. Churchill Livingstone, Edinburgh, pp 12–28
84. Oestrup LT, Fredrickson JM (1974) Distant transfer of a free living bone graft by microvascular anastomosis. Plast Reconstr Surg 54:274–285
85. Östrup LT et al (1986) The UNILINK instrument system for fast and safe microvascular anastomosis. Ann Plast Surg 17:521–525
86. Pei G et al (2000) A preliminary report of two cases of human hand allograft. Zhonghua Yi Xue Za Zhi 80:417
87. Perritt RA (1950) Recent advances in corneal surgery. In Course No. 280, Am Acad Ophthal Otol
88. Reboul H (1935) L'Artériographie des membres et de Aorte abdomínale. Etude critique. Preface de Ch. Laubry. Masson & Cie, Paris
89. Research Laboratory for Replantation of Severed Limb, Shanghai Sixth People's Hospital (1976) Free muscle transplantation by microsurgical neurovascular anastomoses. Report of a case. Chin Med J 2:47–50
90. Rohman M, Goetz RH, Dee R (1960) Double coronary artery-internal mammary artery anastomoses, tantalum ring technique. Surg Forum 11:236–237
91. Salmon PA, Assimacopoulos CA (1964) Microsurgery. Minn Med 47:679
92. Samii H, Wallenberg R (1972) Tier experimentelle untersuchungen uber den einfluss der spannung auf den regenerationserfolg nach nervennaht. Acta Neurochir 27:87–110
93. Schumaker HB, Lowenberg RI (1948) Experimental studies in vascular repair. 1. Comparison of reliability of various methods of end-to-end arterial sutures. Surgery 79:24
94. Siegel B, Acevedo FJ (1962) Vein anastomosis by electrocoaptive union. Surg Forum 13: 233–235
95. Siegel B, Acevedo FJ (1963) Electrocoaptive union of blood vessels: a preliminary experimental study. J Surg Res 3:90–96

96. Smith JW (1964) Microsurgery of peripheral nerves. Plast Reconstr Surg 33:317–329
97. Sterling JA (1959) Experimental use of an apparatus for stapling small blood vessels. J Albert Einstein Med Cent 7:192–193
98. Sterling JA (1964) The use of a simplified stapling apparatus for automatic suturing of small blood vessels. Angiology 15:246–249
99. Strauch B, Bloomberg AE, Lewin MC (1971) An experimental approach to mandibular replacement: island vascular composite rib grafts. Br J Plast Surg 24:334–341
100. Swan H (1950) Resection of thoracic aortic aneurysm using a stored human arterial transplant. Arch Surg 61:732–737
101. Swolin K (1967) Fertilitatsoperationen. 1. Literatur und methodik. Acta Obstet Gynecol Scand 46:234–250
102. Szilagyi DE (1958) The clinical use of an elastic dacron prosthesis. Arch Surg 77:538–551
103. Tamai S, Komatsu S, Sakamoto H et al (1970) Free muscle trans-plants in dogs, with microsurgical neurovascular anastomoses. Plast Reconstr Surg 46:219–225
104. Tamai S, Sasauchi N, Horii Y et al (1972) Microvascular surgery in orthopedics and traumatology. J Bone Joint Surg 54B:637–647
105. Taylor GI, Miller DGH, Ham FJ (1975) The free vascularized bone grafts. A clinical extension of microvascular technique. Plast Reconstr Surg 55:533–544
106. Taylor GI, Watson N (1978) One stage repair of compound leg defects with free, revascularized flaps of groin skin and iliac bone. Plast Reconstr Surg 61:494–506
107. Terzis JK, Faibisoff BA, Williams HB (1975) The nerve gap: suture under tension vs. graft. Plast Reconstr Surg 56:166–170
108. Troutman RC (1965) The operating microscope in ophthalmic surgery. Trans Am Ophthalmol Soc 63:335–348
109. Ueba Y, Fujikawa S (1983) Vascularized fibula grafts to neurofiblomatosis of the ulna-a 9 year follow up. Orthop Surg Traumata (Japan) 26:595–600
110. Vogelfanger IJ, Beattie WG (1958) A concept of automation in vascular surgery: a preliminary report on a mechanical instrument for arterial anastomosis. Can J Surg 1:262
111. Walz W (1959) Sterilitatsoperationen an der tukbe mit hilfe eines operationmikroskope. Z Geburtshilfe Gynek 153:49–55
112. Williams HB, Terzis JK (1976) Single fascicular recordings: an intraoperative diagnostic tool for the management of peripheral nerve lesions. Plast Reconstr Surg 57:562–569
113. Winfrey EW, Foster JH (1962) Prevention of arterial thrombosis with a negatively charged wire suture. Surg Forum 13:229–232
114. Yamano Y (1985) Replantation of the amputated distal part of the fingers. J Hand Surg 10:211–218

History of Telesurgery

2

James Wall and Jacques Marescaux

Hippocrates (480–390 B.C.) defined surgery as the therapeutic activity practiced by the means of the "hands." The figure of the ancient surgeon was surrounded by a kind of mysticism because they touched the inside of the sacred human body with naked hands. The early Greek surgeons reported the use of limited surgical tools to assist with surgical procedures beginning the separation of the surgeon's hands from the patient. Halsted pioneered the use of the surgical glove in 1894 and separated the surgeon a little further form the patient. The twentieth century has seen the addition of laparoscopic surgery that moved the surgeon's hand outside the body to reduce surgical trauma and improve patient outcomes. Despite these advances, some form of physical contact between the surgeon and patient has always remained. Surgical robotics at the turn of the twenty-first century has produced the technology to disrupt even the paradigm of surgeon-patient proximity.

Robotics entered the operating room in 1985 with the PUMA 200 industrial robot adapted for CT-guided brain biopsy [5]. In 1988, the PROBOT was an ultrasound-guided system used to perform prostatic resections [4]. The first commercially available medical robot came in 1992 with the ROBODOC (Integrated Surgical Systems, Sacramento, CA). The system was designed and approved to precisely mill the femur for hip replacements. This first generation of surgical robots was notable for performing image-guided precision tasks but was limited by the need for preoperative planning and basic computer interfaces.

The evolution of surgical robots has led to a current generation of real-time telemanipulators. The AESOP® (Automated Endoscopic System for Optimal Position, Computer Motion Inc., Goleta, CA) was the first robotic system approved for general surgery [1, 9]. In the emerging era of laparoscopy, the system was designed to assist the surgeon by taking control of the laparoscopic camera and responding to voice

---

J. Wall, M.D. • J. Marescaux, M.D., (Hon) F.R.C.S., F.A.C.S., (Hon) J.S.E.S. (✉)
IRCAD, Department of General, Digestive and Endocrine Surgery,
University Hospital of Strasbourg, 1 place de l'Hôpital, Strasbourg 67091, France
e-mail: jacques.marescaux@ircad.fr

P. Liverneaux et al. (eds.), *Telemicrosurgery*,
DOI 10.1007/978-2-8178-0391-3_2, © Springer-Verlag France 2013

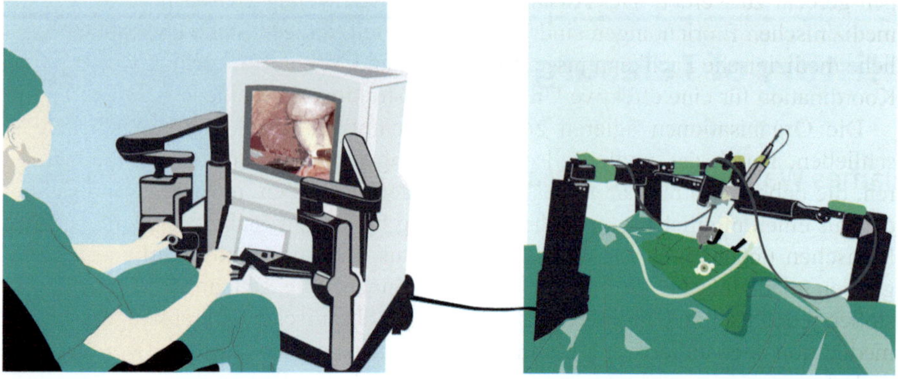

Fig. 2.1 The fundamental configuration of a surgical robot that enables telesurgery. The surgeon and control panel are separated from the patient and robotic arms

commands [8, 11, 14, 15]. The next step was to create telemanipulation machines where the robot mimics the gestures of the surgeon (Fig. 2.1). In these units, the "master" control console, from which the surgeon operates, is physically separated from the "slave" unit, composed of the robotic arms performing surgery on the patient.

The development of telesurgery arose in the 1970s with the aim to replace the surgeon physical presence in situations of mass casualties in hostile environments such as war or natural catastrophes. While the foundation of telemanipulation surgical systems can be traced back to the United States National Aeronautics and Space Administration (NASA), their major development was funded by DARPA (Defense Advanced Research Project Administration) as a potential military tool for remote surgical care of the injured soldier. Two main teleoperator surgical robots were developed from the research: the da Vinci® Surgical System (Intuitive Surgical, Inc., Sunnyvale, CA) and the ZEUS® system (Computer Motion, Goleta, CA). Intuitive Surgical and Computer Motion merged in 2003, resulting in a single FDA-approved robotic platform on the market today that carries the name da Vinci®.

Early systems required the surgeon to be in the same room as the patient. However, with the use of telecommunications, both telementoring and telemanipulation were attempted from remote locations [2, 3]. One early report from 1996 demonstrated the ability of a surgeon in the same city to successfully mentor another surgeon as well as manipulate an endoscopic camera [7]. While successful, it was felt that latency in data transmission limited telemanipulation to a distance of a few hundred kilometers [12].

Fortunately, the telecommunications industry has also seen significant improvements since the invention of the telephone in 1876. Modern fiber-optic global connections allow reliable high-bandwidth data transmission with delays of less than 500 ms. The combination of high-speed telecommunications and a modern telemanipulator enabled all limitations on global telesurgery to be broken by "Operation Lindberg," the first transatlantic surgical procedure. Using advanced asynchronous transfer mode (ATM) telecommunication technology, a surgeon

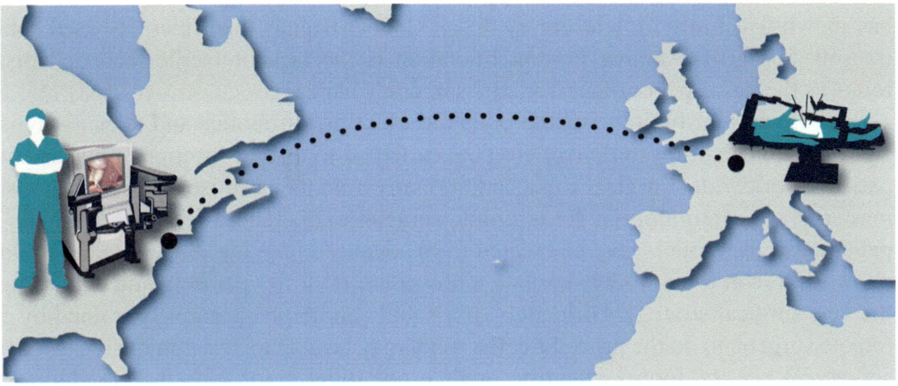

Fig. 2.2 Operation Lindberg: the first transcontinental telesurgical procedure

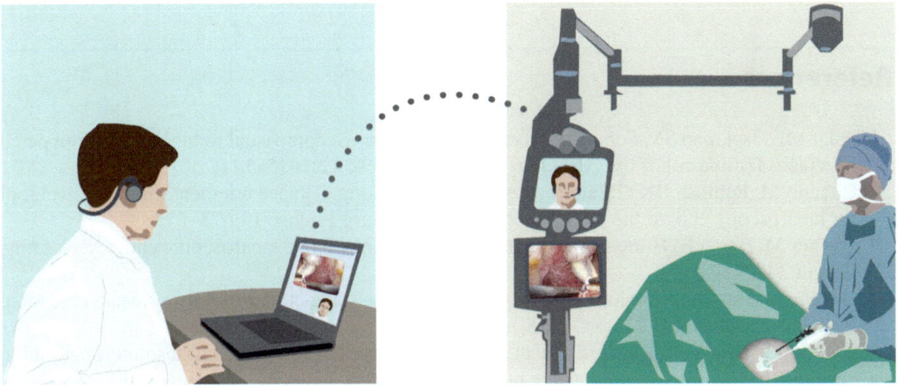

Fig. 2.3 Surgical telementoring enables a specialist surgeon to remotely assist in complex procedures

worked from a control panel in New York, United States, to successfully perform a complete cholecystectomy on a patient in Strasbourg, France (Fig. 2.2) [6].

The routine use of telesurgical applications is still under development. In addition to technical challenges, there are many medical-legal, billing, and liability issues that must be resolved to enable telesurgery across state and national boundaries. Progress has been made in telementoring, where specialist surgeons can mentor local surgeons through telepresence. Telementoring programs that allow rural hospitals access to specialists are being established worldwide (Fig. 2.3). Early reports shown that specialist surgical skills can be disseminated effectively using telementoring [13].

Telesurgery remains in its infancy. Significant challenges remain for the field including the cost-effectiveness, access to bandwidth, regulations, and adoption. Telesurgery in extremely remote locations is limited by the availability of advanced telecommunications. However, recently work on satellite-based telecommunications has shown feasibility for telesurgery despite higher latency than Internet-based data transmission [10]. Another current limitation is the lack of tactile feedback that removes the key aspect of feel from the surgeon's hands.

Despite current limitations, the potential of surgical robotics and telesurgery is enormous. The ability to deliver surgical expertise to distant locations will benefit patients worldwide. Surgical robots additionally hold the promise of more than just master–slave configurations for a remote surgeon to operate in real time. One day, patient-specific models may be created from advanced imaging. Such models could allow a surgeon to remotely simulate a procedure prior to operating and determine the best surgical strategy. Ultimately, if a robot can be preoperatively trained by a remote surgeon to do the procedure, the robot may be able to autonomously perform surgery. While the future is hard to predict, one thing is for sure, the paradigm of physical contact between the surgeon and patient has been broken leading to an era where surgeons can operate from across the room, across the country, and even across continents.

References

1. Allaf ME, Jackman SV, Schulam PG et al (1998) Laparoscopic visual field. Voice vs foot pedal interfaces for control of the AESOP robot. Surg Endosc 12:1415–1418
2. Cubano M, Poulose BK, Talamini MA et al (1999) Long distance telementoring. A novel tool for laparoscopy aboard the USS Abraham Lincoln. Surg Endosc 13:673–678
3. Gagner M, Begin E, Hurteau R et al (1994) Robotic interactive laparoscopic cholecystectomy. Lancet 343:596–597
4. Harris SJ, Arambula-Cosio F et al (1988) The Probot – an active robot for prostate resection. Proc Inst Mech Eng H 211:317–325
5. Kwoh YS, Hou J, Jonckheere EA et al (1988) A robot with improved absolute positioning accuracy for CT guided stereotactic brain surgery. IEEE Trans Biomed Eng 35:153–160
6. Marescaux J, Leroy J, Gagner M et al (2001) Transatlantic robot-assisted telesurgery. Nature 27:379–380
7. Moore RG, Adams JB, Partin AW et al (1996) Telementoring of laparoscopic procedures: initial clinical experience. Surg Endosc 10:107–110
8. Nebot PB, Jain Y, Haylett K et al (2003) Comparison of task performance of the camera-holder robots EndoAssist and Aesop. Surg Laparosc Endosc Percutan Tech 13:334–338
9. Omote K, Feussner H, Ungeheuer A et al (1999) Self-guided robotic camera control for laparoscopic surgery compared with human camera control. Am J Surg 177:321–324
10. Rayman R, Croome K, Galbraith N et al (2007) Robotic telesurgery: a real-world comparison of ground- and satellite-based internet performance. Int J Med Robot 3:111–116
11. Sackier JM, Wang Y (1994) Robotically assisted laparoscopic surgery. From concept to development. Surg Endosc 8:63–66
12. Satava RM (1999) Emerging technologies for surgery in the 21st century. Arch Surg 134:1197–1202
13. Schlachta CM, Lefebvre KL, Sorsdahl AK et al (2010) Mentoring and telementoring leads to effective incorporation of laparoscopic colon surgery. Surg Endosc 24:841–844
14. Unger SW, Unger HM, Bass RT (1994) AESOP robotic arm. Surg Endosc 8:1131
15. Wagner AA, Varkarakis IM, Link RE et al (2006) Comparison of surgical performance during laparoscopic radical prostatectomy of two robotic camera holders, EndoAssist and AESOP: a pilot study. Urology 68:70–74

Description of Robots

3

Jesse Creed Selber

3.1 Introduction

Since the dawn of Western civilization, robotic concepts have been a part of humanity (Table 3.1). The ancient Greeks described a variety of "automata," or semiautonomous systems. Leonardo da Vinci first described humanoid robots during the Enlightenment. The word "robot" seems to have been first penned by the Czeck writer, Karel Čapek in his play, *R.U.R.* (*Rossum's Universal Robots*), published in 1920 [1]. In the 1950 collection, *I, Robot*, Isaac Asimov coined the term "Robotics" and authored the "Three Laws," intended to govern the activity of conscious robots. Since that time, human-like robots have continued to ignite our imagination, appearing throughout the modern history of science fiction – from the *Forbidden Planet's* Robby the Robot and *Star Wars'* R2D2 and C3PO to the cartoon robots Rosie of the *Jetson's* and Bender of *Futurama*; from the murderous robots, HAL (2001) and the Terminator to Pixar's lovable WALL-E and EVE (Fig. 3.1). In many ways, we have imagined these robots as sentient beings, created in our own various images – complete with the ability to exhibit judgment, decision making, emotions, and other forms of agency restricted to the human mind.

While artificial intelligence of this sort is far from a reality, robots do play a crucial role in our everyday lives. The engineering definition of a robot is "an electro-mechanical intelligent agent that can perform tasks either autonomously or semiautonomously." In contemporary society, there are two main types of robots. The first is the preprogrammed robot, which performs a task or series of tasks again and again, exactly same way each time. These robots have replaced human hands with the precise and tireless movements of machines on most assembly lines (Fig. 3.2). Our automobiles, electronics, microprocessors, and many more of our

J.C. Selber, M.D., M.P.H.
Department of Plastic Surgery – Unit 1488, M.D. Anderson Cancer Center,
University of Texas, 1400 Pressler St, Houston, TX 77030, USA
e-mail: jcselber@manderson.org

P. Liverneaux et al. (eds.), *Telemicrosurgery*,
DOI 10.1007/978-2-8178-0391-3_3, © Springer-Verlag France 2013

Table 3.1 Timeline of robotic history

Date	Significance	Name	Inventor
First century	Descriptions of over a hundred machines and automata, including a fire engine, wind organ, coin-operated machine, and steam-powered aeolipile, in *Pneumatica* and *Automata* by Heron		Ctesibius, Philo, Heron, and others
1206	Early programmable automata	Robot band	Al-Jazari
1495	Designs for a humanoid robot	Mechanical knight	Leonardo da Vinci
1738	Mechanical duck that was able to eat, flap its wings, and excrete	Digesting Duck	Jacques de Vaucanson
Nineteenth century	Japanese mechanical toys that served tea, fired arrows, and painted	*Karakuri* toys	Hisashige Tanaka
1921	First fictional automata called "robots" appear in the play *R.U.R.*	Rossum's Universal Robots	Karel Čapek
1928	Humanoid robot, based on a suit of armor with electrical actuators, exhibited at the annual exhibition of the Model Engineers Society in London	Eric	W. H. Richards
1930s	Humanoid robot exhibited at the 1939 and 1940 World's Fairs	Elektro	Westinghouse Electric Corporation
1948	Simple robots exhibiting biological behaviors	Elsie and Elmer	William Grey Walter
1956	First commercial robot, from the Unimation company founded by George Devol and Joseph Engelberger, based on Devol's patents	Unimate	George Devol
1961	First installed industrial robot	Unimate	George Devol
1963	First palletizing robot	Palletizer	Fuji Yusoki Kogyo
1973	First robot with six electromechanically driven axes	Famulus	KUKA Robot Group
1975	Programmable universal manipulation arm, a Unimation product	PUMA	Victor Scheinman

most valuable assets are produced without a bead of sweat, or a breath of air. Although these preprogrammed robots are perfect for assembly, they are very poorly suited to surgery, because each operative procedure is in some way unique, requiring hundreds of decisions by the surgeon.

The next type of robot, far less common, is based on a command-control platform. Rather than being preprogrammed to perform a defined function, these robots are remotely controlled, in real time, by human beings. NASA's space arm is the prototypical example. This giant robotic extremity is used to perform a variety of tasks in and around the space station, under direct control of experienced astronauts (Fig. 3.3). What makes this type of robot special is that it combines the executive functions of the human mind with the precision of a machine. This is the ideal

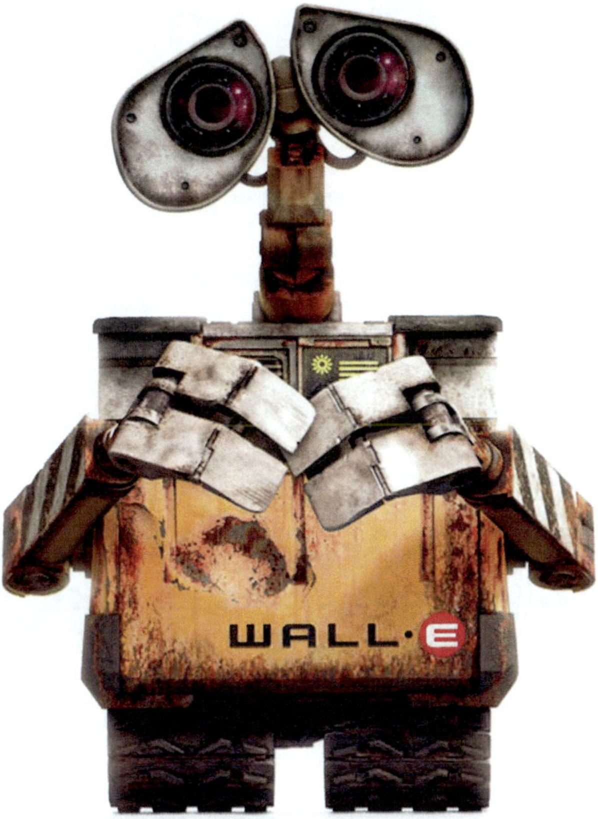

Fig. 3.1 Since the 1940s, public fascination with robots has been manifested in science fiction. Shown here is WALL-E, from Pixar's 2008 animated film about an artificial intelligence robot

system for robotic surgery, since the experience, judgment, and expertise of the surgeon can be channeled through a machine that is unlimited by the constraints of human motor function. The da Vinci® surgical robot is one such system.

3.2 da Vinci® Robot

At the time of the publication of this book, the only clinically available surgical robots are the da Vinci®, da Vinci S®, and da Vinci Si® Surgical Systems and EndoWrist Instruments and Accessories, made by Intuitive Surgical®. The da Vinci Surgical Systems (Models IS1200, 1S2000, 1IS3000) consist of two integrated subsystems: a surgeon console and a patient-side cart (Fig. 3.4). While seated at the surgeon console, the surgeon controls all aspects of the procedure, including movement of the endoscopic instruments and endoscope within the operative field.

The endoscopic instrument and camera movements are controlled by the surgeon through use of the master tool manipulators (MTM), two hand-operated mechanisms residing within the surgeon console (Fig. 3.5). The endoscopic instruments

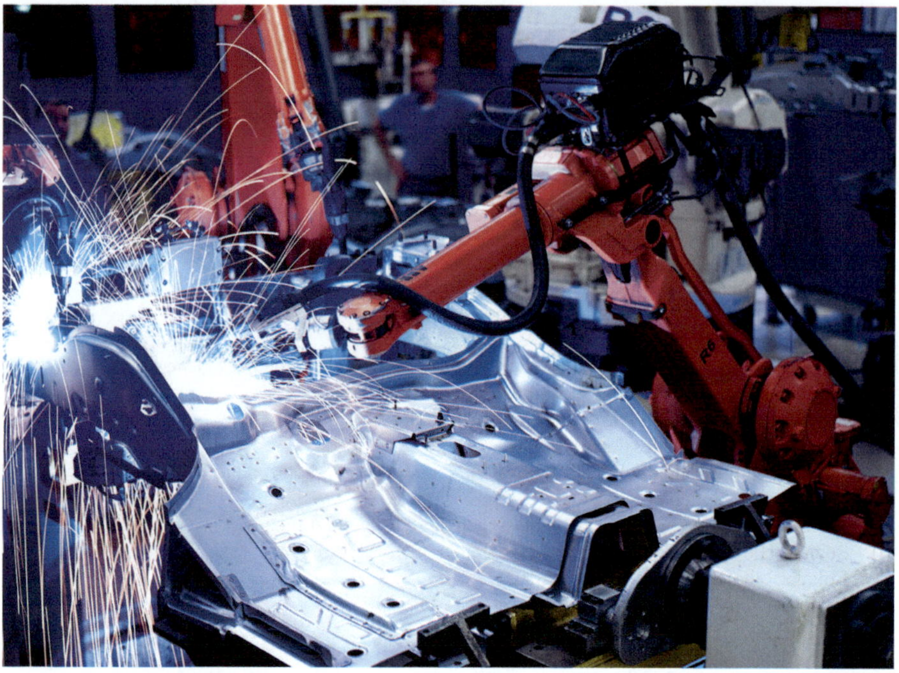

Fig. 3.2 Robots play a huge part in contemporary manufacturing. Preprogrammed robots that repeatedly perform an identical task have replaced humans in most complex assembly line procedures

are held in a fixed position with respect to the patient by either two (or optionally three) unique arms known as patient-side manipulators (PSM), which are located on the patient-side cart (PSC) (Fig. 3.6). The endoscope is also held in a fixed position (with respect to the patient) by another arm, similar to the PSM, known as the endoscope camera manipulator (ECM), which is also located on the PSC. Commands from the surgeon console are relayed to the PSC, which is located immediately adjacent to the patient, via cables. Instrument and endoscope changes are performed by another individual positioned adjacent to the PSC.

The endoscopic vision system used with the da Vinci Surgical Systems, also known as Intuitive Surgical "Insite" Vision System, consists of a stereo endoscope, endoscopic camera, and various accessories, including a light source and light guides (Fig. 3.7). The "Insite" Vision System provides two independent images that are relayed to the surgeon located at the surgeon console, where they are fused to form a 3-D (or alternatively a 2-D image) image of the surgical field. The Intuitive Surgical Endoscopic Instrument Control Systems (da Vinci®, da Vinci S®, and da

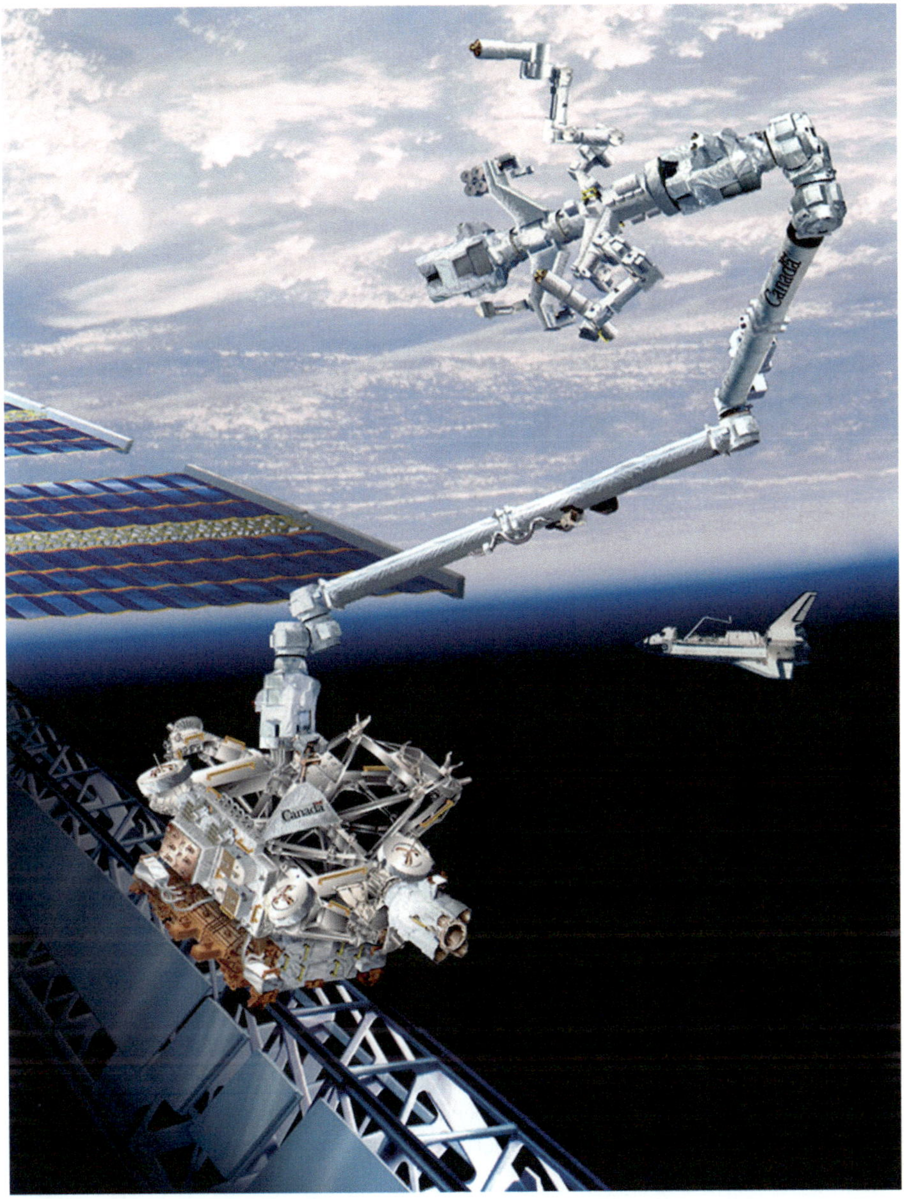

Fig. 3.3 Robots that are controlled in real time by humans are relatively unusual. NASA's space arm is the prototypical example. This giant robotic extremity is used to perform a variety of tasks in and around space stations, under direct control of experienced astronauts. The surgical robot is the type of command and control system

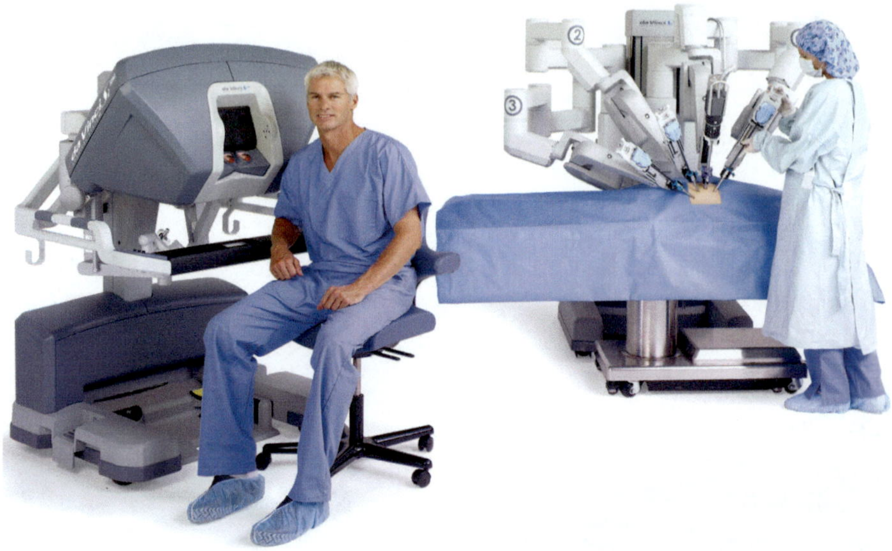

Fig. 3.4 The da Vinci Surgical Systems (Models IS1200, 1S2000, 1IS3000) consist of two integrated subsystems: a surgeon console and a patient-side cart. While seated at the surgeon console, the surgeon controls all aspects of the procedure, including movement of the endoscopic instruments and endoscope within the operative field

Vinci SI® Surgical Systems Models IS1200, 1S2000, 1S3000) are intended to assist in the accurate control of Intuitive Surgical EndoWrist Instruments (Fig. 3.8) and Accessories including rigid endoscopes, blunt and sharp endoscopic dissectors, scissors, scalpels, ultrasonic/harmonic shears, forceps/pickups, needle holders, endoscopic retractors, stabilizers, electrocautery, and accessories (Fig. 3.9) for endoscopic manipulation of tissue, including grasping, cutting, blunt and sharp dissection, approximation, ligation, electrocautery, suturing, delivery and placement of microwave ablation probes and accessories, during urologic surgical procedures, general laparoscopic surgical procedures, gynecologic laparoscopic surgical procedures, transoral otolaryngology surgical procedures restricted to benign and malignant tumors, general thoracoscopic surgical procedures, and thoracoscopically assisted cardiotomy procedures. The system can also be employed with adjunctive mediastinotomy to perform coronary anastomosis during cardiac revascularization.

Because of the utility of this system, robots have found uses in virtually every surgical subspecialty, from urology to cardiac surgery, general surgery to gynecology, and, more recently, ear nose and throat, orthopedics, and plastic surgery. As robotic technology continues to evolve to keep pace with clinical demands, surgical robots will play an ever more prominent role in the lives of both surgeon and patient.

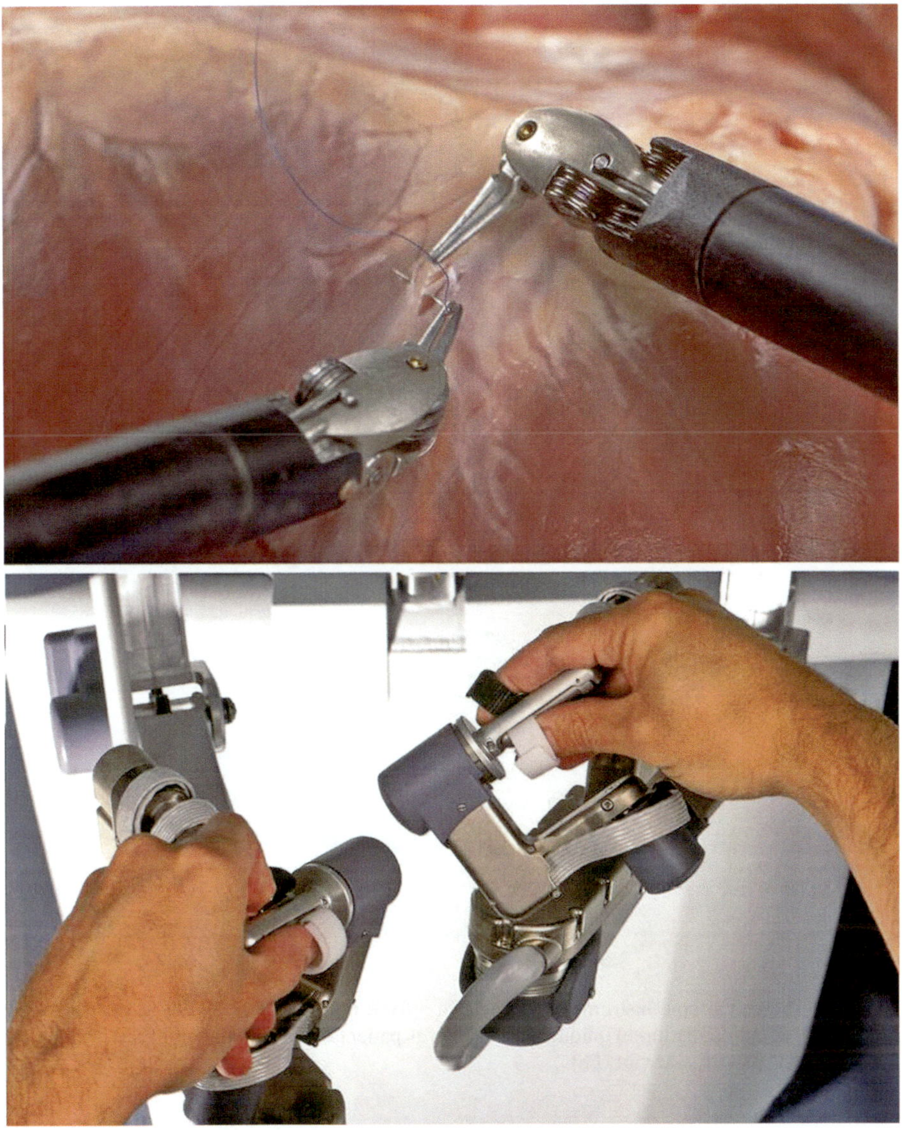

Fig. 3.5 The endoscopic instrument and camera movements are controlled by the surgeon through use of the master tool manipulators (MTM), two hand-operated mechanisms residing within the surgeon console

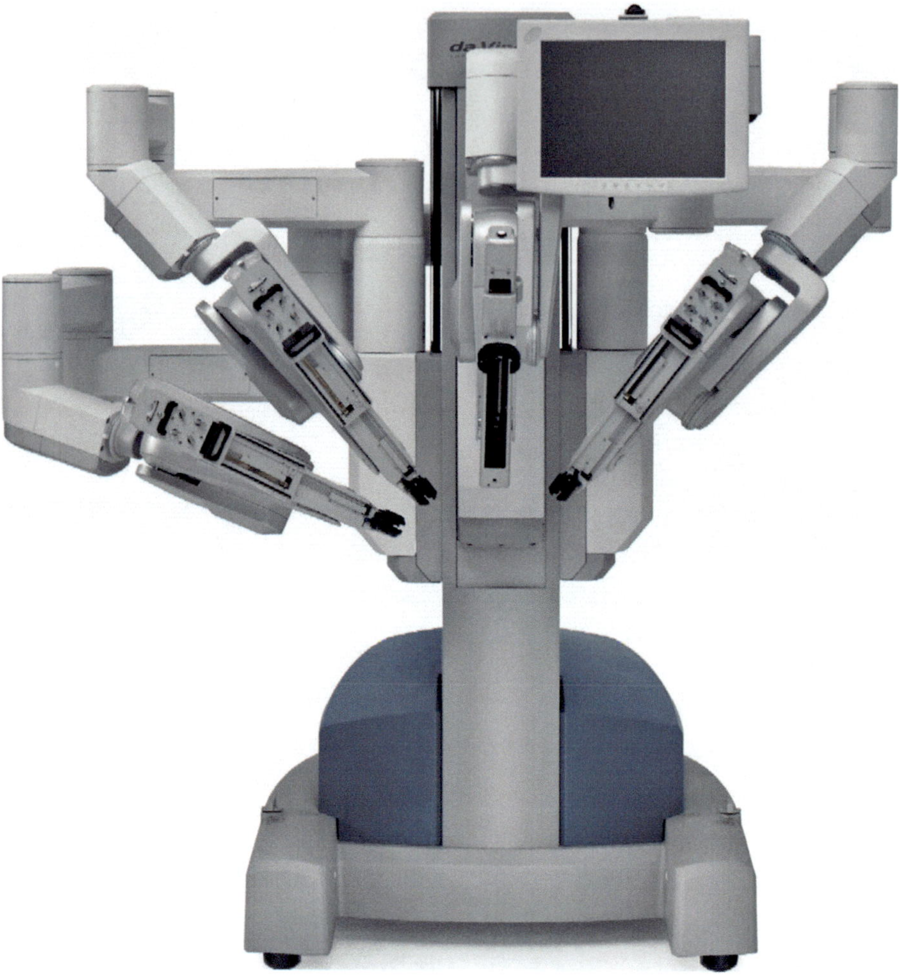

Fig. 3.6 The endoscopic instruments are held in a fixed position with respect to the patient by either two (or optionally three) unique arms known as patient-side manipulators (PSM), which are located on the patient-side cart (PSC)

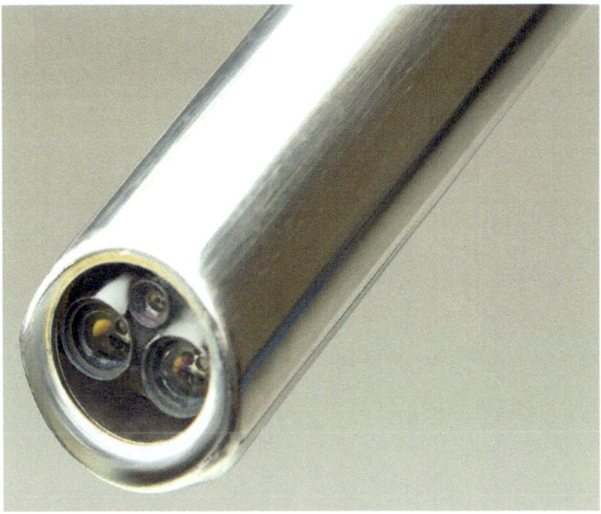

Fig. 3.7 The endoscopic vision system used with the da Vinci Surgical Systems, also known as Intuitive Surgical *Insite* Vision System, consists of a stereo endoscope, endoscopic camera, and various accessories, including a light source and light guides. The *Insite* Vision System provides two independent images that are relayed to the surgeon located at the surgeon console, where they are fused to form a 3-D (or alternatively a 2-D image) image of the surgical field

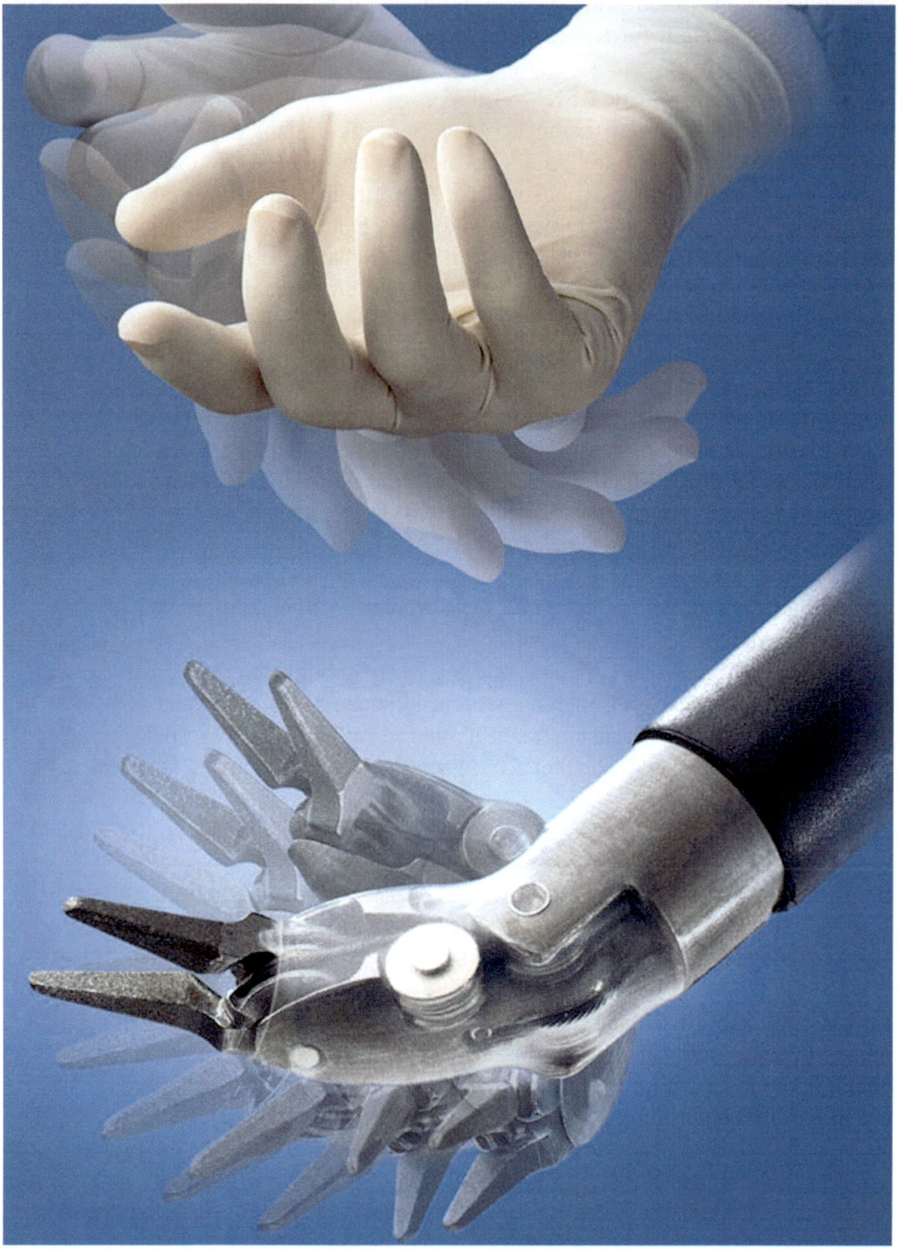

Fig. 3.8 Instrument Control Systems (da Vinci®, da Vinci S®, and da Vinci SI® Surgical Systems Models IS1200, 1S2000, 1S3000) are intended to assist in the accurate control of Intuitive Surgical EndoWrist Instruments and Accessories. Instruments are capable of flexion, extension, supination, pronation, and in most cases grasping, making their movements very analogous to those of the human hand

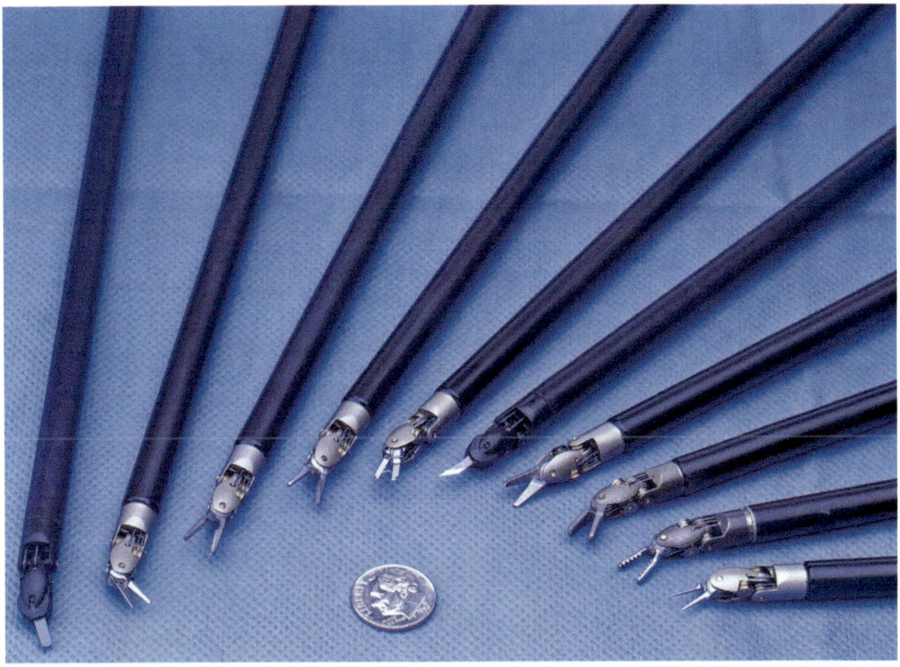

Fig. 3.9 Instruments and accessories include rigid blunt and sharp endoscopic dissectors, scissors, scalpels, ultrasonic/harmonic shears, forceps/pickups, needle holders, endoscopic retractors, stabilizers, electrocautery, and accessories for endoscopic manipulation of tissue, including grasping, cutting, blunt and sharp dissection, approximation, ligation, electrocautery, suturing, delivery and placement of microwave ablation probes and accessories, during urologic surgical procedures, general laparoscopic surgical procedures, gynecologic laparoscopic surgical procedures, transoral otolaryngology surgical procedures restricted to benign and malignant tumors, general thoracoscopic surgical procedures, and thoracoscopically assisted cardiotomy procedures

Conclusion

Robots occupy a special place in the human imagination and a pivotal role in our everyday lives. There is a large gap between the artificial intelligence model about which we fantasize and the task-oriented systems that dominate manufacturing. Surgical robots represent a unique type of robotic system: one that is directed in real time by human hands. This type of interface is ideal for surgery because it combines the executive functions of the surgeon's mind with the precision of a machine.

Reference

1. Zunt D (2007) Who did actually invent the word "robot" and what does it mean? The Karel Čapek website http://capek.misto.cz/english/robot.html. Retrieved 11 Sept 2007

Instruments

4

Sijo Joseph Parekatti and Michael Moran

4.1 Introduction

The history of robotics in surgery is rich and diverse [7]. From the earliest beginnings, there has been continued development of instrumentation to assist the microsurgeon. This chapter will focus on the evolution and development of robot-assisted instrumentation in microsurgery. An understanding of the evolution of our instrumentation may assist us in the further development of robotic tools for the future.

4.2 History of Robotic Instrumentation

4.2.1 1961: Unimate

Isaac Asimov first used the word "robotics" in a short story, "Runaround," published in 1942. One of the first robots Asimov wrote about was a robotherapist – a communication liaison device between man and machine. In 1956, a historic meeting occurred between George C. Devol, a successful inventor and entrepreneur, and engineer Joseph F. Engelberger. Over cocktails, the two discussed the writings of Isaac Asimov. They formulated the beginnings of the first commercially viable robot. They persuaded Norman Schafler of Condec Corporation in Danbury to invest in their venture. Engelberger started the first commercial company to make robots called Unimation (universal automation). Devol wrote the necessary patents. Their first robot was called the "Unimate." This resulted in Engelberger being called the "father of robotics." The first Unimate was installed at a General Motors plant to work with heated die-casting machines. The goal of Unimate was to complete tasks

S.J. Parekatti, M.D. (✉) • M. Moran, M.D.
Urology Department, Winter Haven Hospital, University of Florida,
200 Avenue F, N.E., Winter Haven 33881, FL, USA
e-mail: sijo.parekattil@winterhavenhospital.org

P. Liverneaux et al. (eds.), *Telemicrosurgery*,
DOI 10.1007/978-2-8178-0391-3_4,

that would be considered otherwise unsafe and difficult for humans to perform. Most Unimates were used for die-casting extractions. They were also utilized for spot welding on autobodies. Such tasks were considered particularly hateful jobs for humans. The use of the Unimate for these applications was a huge commercial success. The robots worked reliably and saved money by replacing manual labor.

This was the beginning of a very productive robotic industrial revolution that spawned the modern usage of robots in many of our factories. The Unimate was applied to a variety of other tasks, such as loading and unloading machine tools. Ultimately Westinghouse acquired Unimation, and the entrepreneurs' dream of wealth was achieved. Unimation is still in production today, with robots for sale. The robot idea was hyped to the skies and became high fashion among senior management. Chief executive officers of large corporations bought them, for about $100,000 each, just to put into laboratories to "see what they could do" [5]. In fact, these sales constituted a large part of the robot market. Some companies even reduced their return on investment criteria for investment for robots to encourage their use.

4.2.2 1980s: Green SRI Telepresence Surgical System

The US Department of Defense had long been interested in the development of front-line methods of improving care to injured soldiers. Life-threatening injuries occurring immediately during battle might be salvageable if surgical care could be instantly instituted. In addition, after George Bush's announcement of the United States' intention of getting a man on Mars, the National Aeronautics and Space Administration (NASA) Ames Research Center began to fund proposals for the eventual need for possible surgical intervention on astronauts remote from a hospital [4]. A team of investigators led by Michael McGreevey and Stephen Ellis began to investigate 19861 computer-generated scenarios that could be perceived on head-mounted displays (HMDs) [2]. To this team, eventually came Scott Fisher who added 3D audio and came up with the concept of "telepresence." This was the notion that one person could be projected with the immersive experience of another (real or imaginary). Joseph Rosen, a plastic surgeon at Stanford University, began to experiment with Philip Green from Stanford Research Institute (SRI) to develop dexterity-enhancing robots for telemanipulation [3]. These two teams would eventually collaborate, and together Joe Rosen and Scott Fisher produced the fundamentals of telepresence surgery. This combined the dexterity-enhancing robotics of Green and the "virtual reality" systems of NASA for an immersive surgical experience. The initial systems conceived that the surgeon would be in a helmeted immersive sight/sound environment wired electronically to "data gloves" that would digitally tract the surgeon's motions and reproduce them at remote robotic instruments. The notion of the data glove came from Jaron Lanier, a computer scientist interested in virtual reality. The initial targeted surgery was on the hand and vascular anastomosis.

Many of the initially designed features of Green's telepresence system were at the time unworkable from an engineering standpoint. The HMD was subsequently replaced with monitors, and the data gloves were replaced with handles for controllers at the surgeon's console. Since the imperative at this time was for space and/or military application for acute surgical care, the end-effectors were substantially similar to open surgical instruments. This was all occurring in the late 1980s. By 1989, then Colonel Richard Satava stationed at Silas B. Hayes Army Hospital in Monterey became involved in this project, and more federal aid became available. Serendipitously, that same year found Jacques Perrisat of Bordeaux presenting on the technique of laparoscopic cholecystectomy at the Society of American Gastrointestinal Endoscopic Surgeons (SAGES) in Atlanta. Upon returning from this meeting, the team of investigators began to consider developing a system that could be applied to minimally invasive laparoscopic surgery. Satava presented a videotape of a bowel anastomosis using the telepresence surgery system to the Association of Military Surgeons of the United States. The results of this single demonstration of this technology resulted in a July 1992 Defense Advanced Research Projects Agency (DARPA) grant for further investigation and development. In addition, Satava became the program manager for Advance Biomedical Technologies to aid funding of technologically advanced projects. With the funding now possible, by 1995, the robotic system was in prototype mounted into an armored vehicle (the Bradley 557A) that could "virtually" take the surgeon to the front lines and immediately render surgical care to the wounded, called MEDFAST (Medical Forward Area Surgical Team) [8]. The technology caught the attention of Alan Alda (aka Hawkeye Pierce from the TV drama M*A*S*H), now the voice of Discovery Channel that filmed a piece on this technology.

4.2.3 1993: HERMES and AESOP

In 1993, Yulyn Wang, Ph.D. from the University of California, Santa Barbara, developed software for control motion of robotic systems and founded a company called Computer Motion. Wang succeeded in developing a robotic camera holder called Automated Endoscopic System for Optimal Positioning (AESOP). He became interested in complete robotic surgery and obtained DARPA (Defense Advanced Research Projects Agency) funding and money from entrepreneurs to develop ZEUS, a modular robotic system to be integrated with AESOP. HERMES was the integrated operating room control system that allowed the complete integration of Computer Motion's robotic system [9]. In 2001, a device combining both the AESOP and HERMES was developed by Computer Motion, the ZEUS robotic system. This was a master–slave device that allowed the surgeon to be positioned at a console and control a separate robotic slave device.

4.2.4 1995–2000: da Vinci Surgical System

In 1995, Frederic H. Moll, M.D. (a successful entrepreneur), Rob Younge (an engineer), and John Freund (an MBA from Harvard) became interested in the potential of the "telepresence" work from SRI. They created a start-up company called Intuitive Surgical [6]. The device comprised of three main components: (1) a master–slave software-driven system that provided control of seven-degree-of-freedom robotic instruments, (2) a 3D immersive vision system, and (3) a sensor-based safety monitoring system to continuously reassess the device's performance to maximize patient safety.

The first prototype was tested in March of 1997. By April 15, 1997, the first robotic surgery was performed by Jacques Himpens and Guy Cardiere of Brussels, Belgium: a robotic cholecystectomy [4]. The first 200-patient trial was completed on cholecystectomy and Nissen fundoplications leading to Food and Drug Administration (FDA) approval of this robotic system in July 2000. In December 2002, the FDA also approved the use of the next generation da Vinci System with the addition of a fourth robotic arm to the tower. The use of the robot in urology rapidly advanced with applications in prostatectomy, nephrectomy, partial nephrectomy, and cystectomy.

4.3 Current Robotic Surgical Platform and Applications

Intuitive Surgical (Sunnyvale, CA) now offers an enhanced 4-arm da Vinci type Si robotic system with high-definition digital visual magnification that allows for greater magnification than the standard robotic system (up to 10–15×). The enhanced magnification capability allows the surgeon to position the camera 6–7 cm away from the operative field to avoid any local tissue effects from the heat emitted from the camera lighting (this was a problem with the older system, where the camera had to place within 2–3 cm of the operative field for microsurgery). This new system allows greater range of motion and better microsurgical instrument handling. The additional fourth arm has improved range of motion and positioning capabilities to provide the microsurgeon with one additional tool during procedures. The new "Si" system also allows for dual surgeons to operate via dual consoles that may control one robotic system. This allows a primary surgeon to guide a trainee surgeon through robotic procedures.

4.4 New Robotic Microsurgical Advances

The da Vinci platform is now being utilized for robot-assisted microsurgical procedures in urology such as vasectomy reversal, subinguinal varicocelectomy, and denervation of the spermatic cord. The platform is used to complete the microsurgical components of the surgery in lieu of an operating microscope. There are a few enhancements and devices that have been developed that may take robotic microsurgical applications further. These are presented below.

4.4.1 Current Robotic Microsurgical Instruments

The standard robotic microsurgical instruments currently available are Black Diamond Micro Forceps (Fig. 4.1), Micro Bipolar Forceps (Fig. 4.2), Potts Scissor

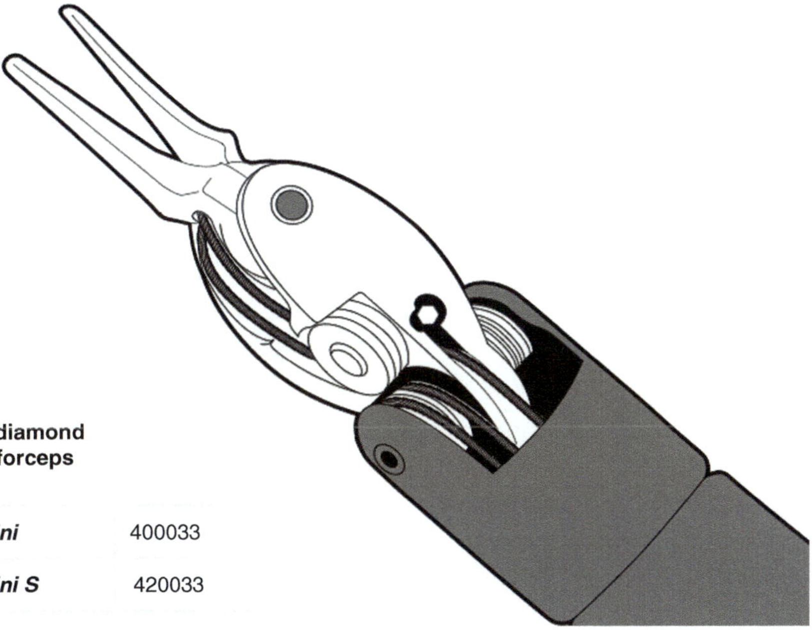

Black diamond micro forceps

da vicini	400033
da vicini S	420033

Fig. 4.1 Black diamond micro forceps

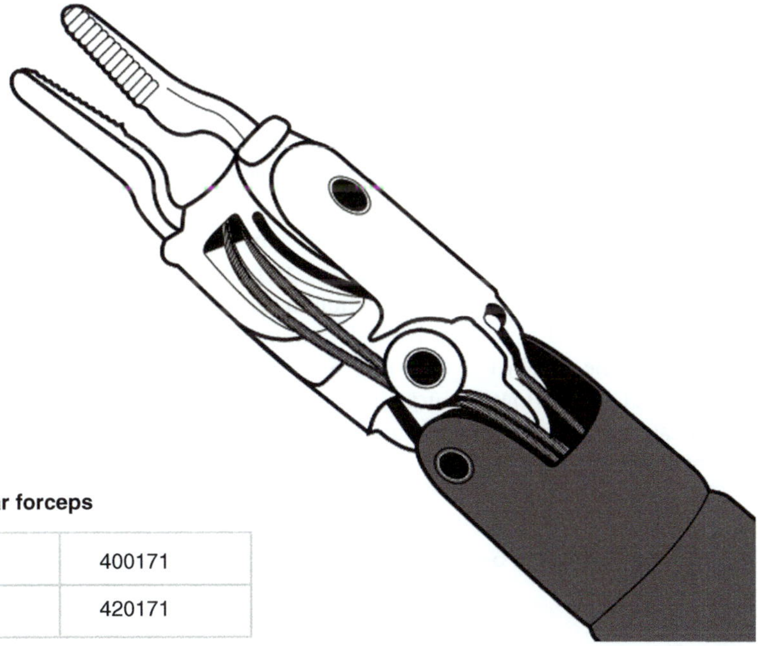

Micro bipolar forceps

da vinci	400171
da vinci S	420171

Fig. 4.2 Micro bipolar forceps

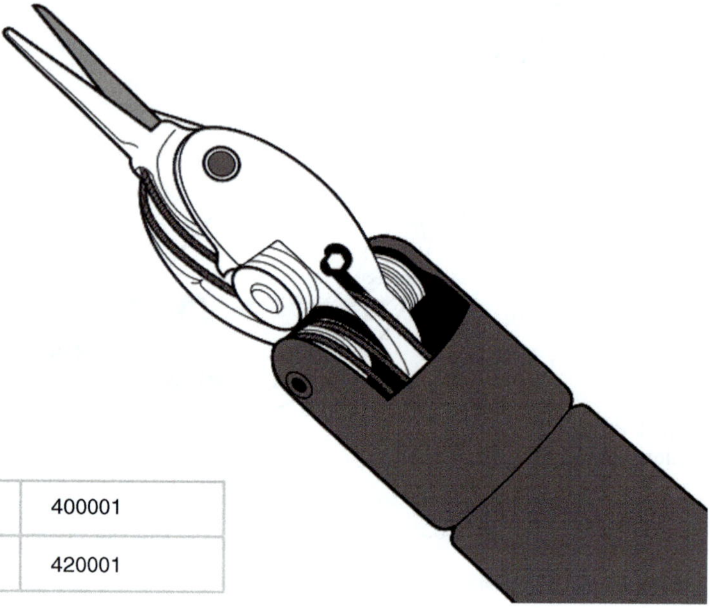

Potts scissors

da vinci	400001
da vinci S	420001

Fig. 4.3 Potts scissor

(Fig. 4.3), Curved Monopolar Scissor (Fig. 4.4), and the Snap-fit Blade (Fig. 4.5). These instruments have been successfully utilized to perform a number of robot-assisted microsurgical procedures. As utilization increases and more applications are developed, these instruments are likely to further improve.

4.4.2 Enhanced 100× Digital Visual Magnification

The miniaturization and development of advanced digital microscopic cameras (100–250×) allows even greater magnification than the standard robotic (10–15×) and microscopic (10–20×) magnification in use at this time. Our group is currently involved in clinical trials of a 100× digital camera (Digital Inc, China) that can be utilized via the TilePro™ da Vinci S or Si robotic system (Intuitive Surgical, Sunnyvale, CA) to allow the surgeon to toggle or use simultaneous 100× and 10–15× visualization. This provides the surgeon with unparalleled visual acuity for complex microsurgical procedures.

4.4.3 Enhanced 16–18× Optical Magnification Multi-view Platform (VITOM)

One of the caveats of the current robotic platform is the limited 12–15× digital magnification that reveals pixilation when microsurgeons are performing complex

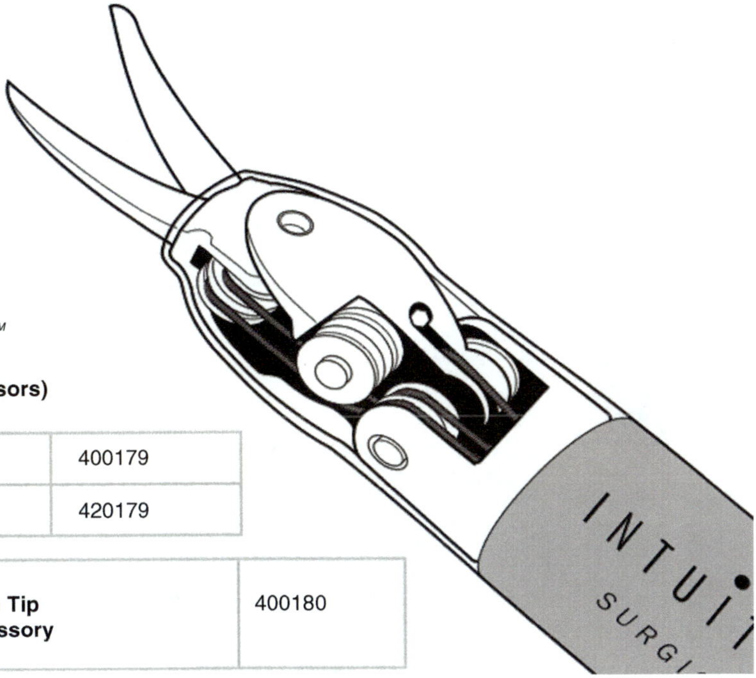

***Hot Shears*™**

(Monopolar curved scissors)

da vinci	400179
da vinci S	420179

Shown With Tip Cover Accessory	400180

Fig. 4.4 Curved monopolar scissors

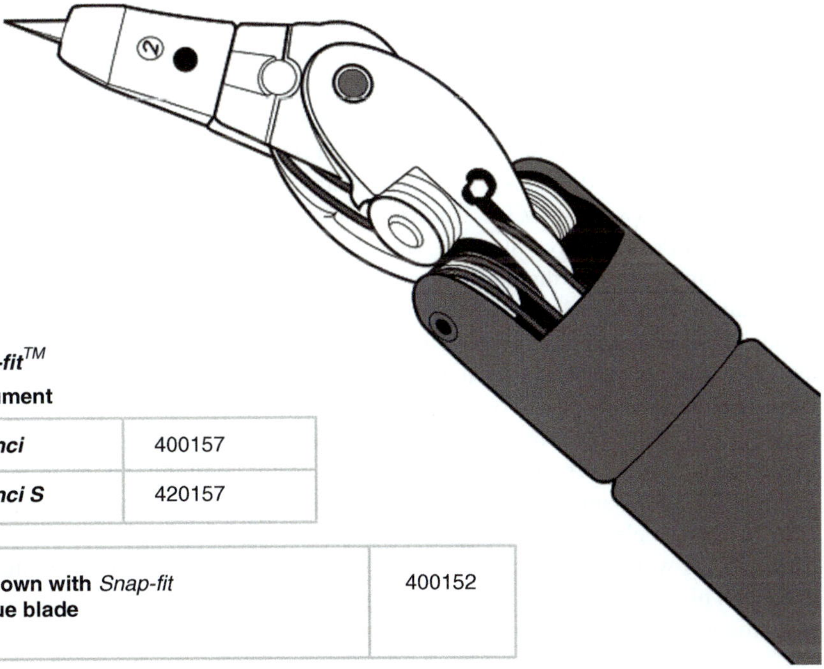

***Snap-fit*™**

Instrument

da Vinci	400157
da Vinci S	420157

Shown with *Snap-fit* blue blade	400152

Fig. 4.5 Snap-fit micro blade

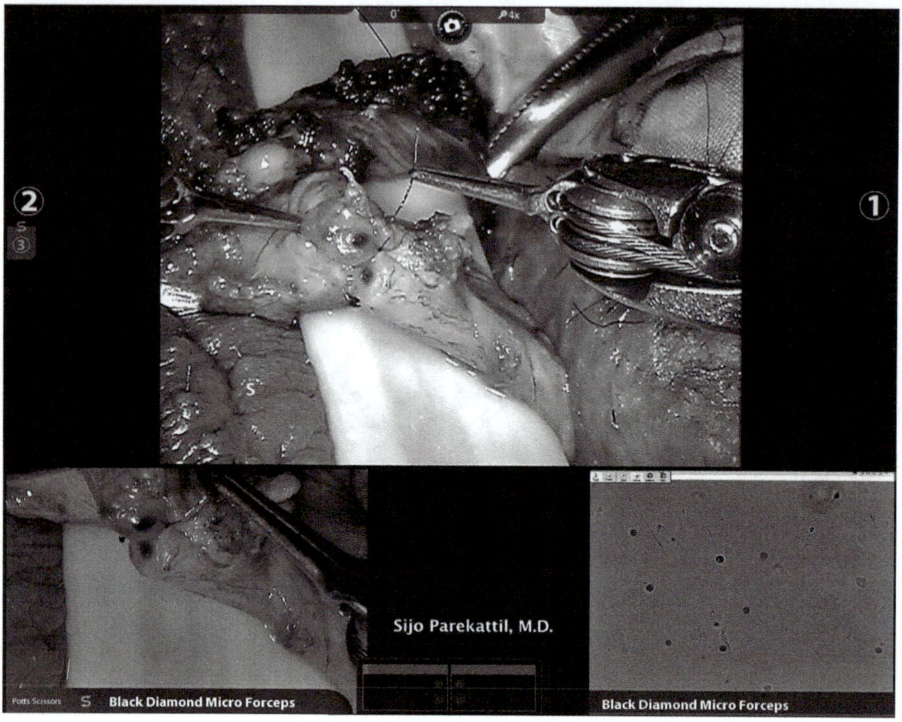

Fig. 4.6 Robot console image using the TilePro™ integration software and the VITOM (Karl Storz Inc.) camera system

reconstructive procedures at higher magnification. We have utilized an enhanced optical high-definition multi-view platform for robot-assisted surgery that provides an additional simultaneous 16–18× optical magnification view for the microsurgeon. We reviewed 86 robot-assisted microsurgical cases performed with this new platform from Dec 2010 to April 2011 by a single microsurgeon.

The VITOM (Karl Storz Inc, Tuttlingen, Germany) imaging system was utilized with the TilePro (Intuitive Surgical, Sunnyvale, CA) robotic surgical console software system to provide three simultaneous real-time video images to the microsurgeon during robot-assisted microsurgery: (1) a 12–15× 3D digital image via the standard robotic camera, (2) a 16–18× optical high-definition view via the VITOM, and (3) a 40× optical microscopic view of fluids being examined by the assistant or laboratory technician (e.g., for vasal, epididymal, or testicular fluid evaluation for sperm). This platform provides the microsurgeon with a cockpit view of all three video inputs in the surgeon console (Figs. 4.6 and 4.7). Eighty-six cases were performed: 26 vasectomy reversals, 43 microsurgical denervation of the spermatic cord, 10 varicocelectomy, and 7 μ TESE (testicular sperm extraction).

All cases were completed successfully without any technical difficulties. The enhanced platform provided the microsurgeon with improved visual acuity at higher magnifications. It also allowed the microsurgeon to perform surgery with a

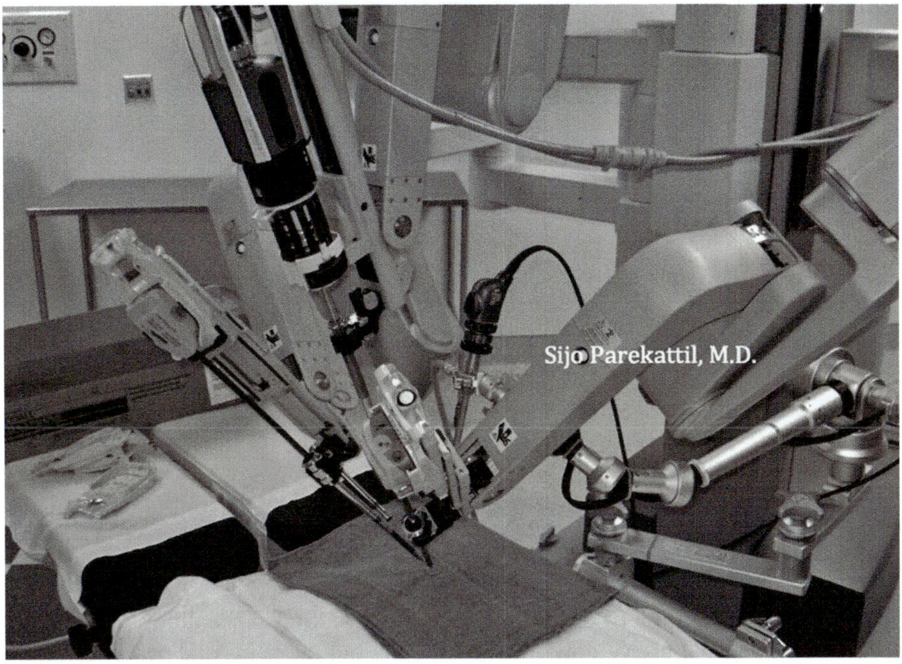

Fig. 4.7 Robotic setup with the additional nitrogen-powered arm for the VITOM camera system (Karl Storz Inc.)

simultaneous view at two differing focal lengths – one showing the overall global view and the other a focused high-definition optical magnification view. This made the procedures more efficient since the surgeon did not have to move the robotic camera in and out to view the field from different focal ranges. This new platform appears to overcome the magnification caveat of the current robotic microsurgical system. However, further evaluation and development is needed.

4.4.4 Robotic Doppler Flow Probe

A recent study by Cocuzza et al. [1] has shown that the systematic use of intraoperative vascular Doppler ultrasound during microsurgical subinguinal varicocelectomy improves precise identification and preservation of testicular blood supply. During robotic microsurgical cases, the standard Doppler probe has to be held by a surgical assistant and cannot be manipulated readily with the robotic graspers. Vascular Technology Inc. (Nashua, NH, USA) has developed a new micro-Doppler flow probe (MDP) designed specifically for use with the robotic platform (Fig. 4.8). This new probe allows for easy manipulation of the probe with the fourth arm and allows the surgeon to perform real-time Doppler monitoring of the testicular artery during cases such as robot-assisted microscopic varicocelectomy (RAVx) and robot-assisted

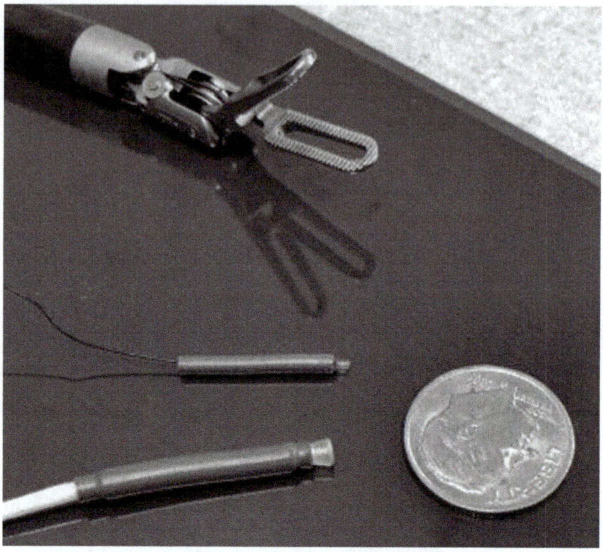

Fig. 4.8 New robotic micro-Doppler probe (Vascular Technology Inc.)

microscopic denervation of the spermatic cord (RMDSC). This allows the surgeon to hear the testicular artery flow while dissecting out the veins and nerves with the other two robotic arms.

To assess this probe, a prospective randomized control trial of the MDP in 273 robotic microsurgical cases from Jul 2009 to Sept 2010 was performed: 67 robotic subinguinal varicocelectomies (RVx) and 206 robotic spermatic cord denervation procedures (RMDSC). The use of the MDP was randomized to 5 RVx and 20 RMDSC procedures. The primary endpoint was the operative time, and secondary endpoint was surgeon ease in testicular artery localization and robotic grasper maneuverability.

The operative duration was not affected by utilization of the MPD ($p=0.5$). The MDP was effective in identifying all testicular arteries within the spermatic cord in all cases. Due to the compact size of the MDP, maneuverability using the robotic grasper was significantly improved over the standard handheld Doppler probe. MDP allowed for full range of motion of the robotic arms allowing the surgeon to easily scan vessels from a wide range of angles. No complications from use of the MDP occurred. The new micro-Doppler probe for robotic microsurgical procedures appears to have performed effectively in this study.

4.4.5 Robot-Assisted Micro-ultrasound Probe (Aloka Inc.)

Aloka Inc. (Wallingford, CT) has recently developed a robotically controlled ultrasound transducer that allows surgeons to obtain full ultrasound imaging with flow mapping (Fig. 4.9). This probe is being modified for robot-assisted microsurgical applications as well.

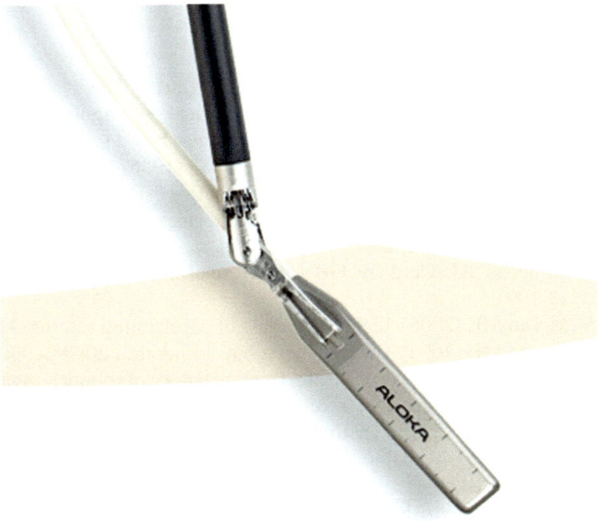

Fig. 4.9 Robotically controlled ultrasound probe (Aloka Inc.)

4.4.6 Micro-hydrodissection Probe (ERBE Inc.)

ERBE Inc. (Atlanta, GA) has developed a micro-hydrodissection probe that can be used in conjunction with their ERBEJET2 pressure adjustable fluid pump. This setup may be used to microdissect through tissue planes and to ligate small-diameter nerve fibers based on specific pressure settings. The use of this device has been found to be beneficial in performing targeted robot-assisted neurolysis or denervation procedures (this study is described in detail in Chap. 19.

4.4.7 Bio-inert or Neuroprotective Wraps (AxoGen Inc.)

AxoGen Inc. (Gainesville, FL) specializes in developing micro-neuroprotective biomaterial wraps (AxoGuard) for use in nerve repair or neurolysis procedures. Studies involving this material are also described in detail in the chapter on Robotic Microsurgery in Urology.

Conclusion

Robotic instrumentation is likely to continue to improve and expand the range of applications in various surgical fields. Robotic applications in a range of areas including microsurgery have the potential to grow. To understand how we will deal with the coming maelstrom of technologic wonders, we could turn to history. Winston Churchill once advised, "The further backwards you look, the further forward you see." The relevance of looking to the foundation of modern robotics is to begin to understand technology and the changes that will affect all aspects of our civilization and not just the way we practice.

References

1. Cocuzza M, Pagani R, Coelho R et al (2010) The systematic use of intraoperative vascular doppler ultrasound during microsurgical subinguinal varicocelectomy improves precise identification and preservation of testicular blood supply. Fertil Steril 93:2396–2399
2. Fisher SS, Humphries J, Robinett W (1986) Virtual environmental display system. In: Proceedings of the workshop on interactive 3-D graphics, Chapel Hill, 1986, vol. 1, pp 1–12
3. Green PS, Satava RM (1991) Telepresence: dexterous procedures in a virtual operating field. Surg Endosc 57:192A
4. Himpens JG, Cardiere GB (1998) Telesurgical laparoscopic cholecystectomy. Surg Endosc 12:1091
5. Moran ME (2006) Technology: law of accelerating returns. J Endourol 20:375–382
6. Moran ME (2006) The da vinci robot. J Endourol 20:986–990
7. RRG Robotic Research Group (2009) History of robotics. Available from: http://www.robotics.utexas.edu/rrg/learn_more/history/ (Accessed on 10 January 2011)
8. Satava RM (2010) History of robotic surgery. The early chronicles: a personal historical perspective. Available from: http://www.websurg.com/robotics/history.php (Accessed on 10 January 2011)
9. Wang Y (1996) Robotically enhanced surgery: from concept to development. Surg Endosc 8:63–66

Robot Installation in Telemicrosurgery 5

Thierry Lequint, Kiyohito Naito, Eric Nectoux,
Sybille Facca, and Philippe Liverneaux

5.1 Introduction

As it is often taught to young residents, an age-old surgical tradition custom says that "a well-installed patient is a well-operated patient" [2]. This saying is all the more meaningful regarding microsurgery and moreover in telemicrosurgery.

T. Lequint, M.D.
Department of Hand Surgery, Strasbourg University Hospitals,
10 Avenue Baumann, F-67403 Illkirch, Strasbourg, France

Department of Orthopeadics, Grand Hôpital,
Charleroi, Belgium

K. Naito, M.D.
Department of Hand Surgery, Strasbourg University Hospitals,
10 Avenue Baumann, F-67403 Illkirch, Strasbourg, France

Department of Orthopeadics, Juntendo University
Tokyo, Japan

E. Nectoux, M.D.
European Institute of TeleSurgery, IRCAD,
F-67000, Strasbourg, France

Department of Children's Surgery and Orthopaedics, Lille University Hospital,
Lille 2 Nord de France University, Lille, France

S. Facca, M.D.
Department of Hand Surgery, Strasbourg University Hospitals,
10 Avenue Baumann F-67403, Illkirch, Strasbourg, France

P. Liverneaux, M.D., Ph.D. (✉)
Department of Hand Surgery, Strasbourg University Hospitals,
10 Avenue Baumann F-67403, Illkirch, Strasbourg, France

European Institute of TeleSurgery, IRCAD,
F-67000, Strasbourg, France
e-mail: philippe.liverneaux@chru-strasbourg.fr

P. Liverneaux et al. (eds.), *Telemicrosurgery*,
DOI 10.1007/978-2-8178-0391-3_5,

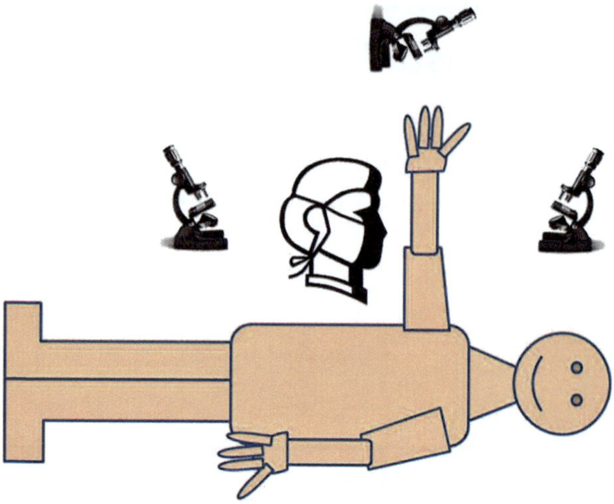

Fig. 5.1 Conventional microsurgical installation. The microsurgeon is seated facing the medial aspect of the forearm. The microscope can be positioned equally well facing the surgeon, at his right- or left-hand side or behind him. Conventional microscope, Surgeon, Robot body, Robot arm, Retractors, Insufflation

Telemicrosurgery requires specific installation, completely different than in conventional microsurgery: robot position with regard to both the patient and the surgeon, surgical approaches, and dissection of and support of a convenient surgical cavity allowing enough space for both camera and surgical instruments to move unimpeded.

5.2 Robot Installation

Installation of the microscope is far easier in conventional microsurgery than in robot in telemicrosurgery.

In conventional microsurgery, the body of the microscope can be installed equally well facing the surgeon, at his right- or left-hand side or behind him (Fig. 5.1). A microscope usually comes with a revolving arm allowing perfect adaptation of the binocular lenses to the surgeon's orbits. The surgeon's forearms lie on adaptive armrests so as to best limit physiological tremor [4].

In telemicrosurgery, the arms of the robot do not extend significantly beyond the robot's body but are aimed instead toward the body, resembling a toreador holding banderillas. Regardless of the surgical field localization, the arms are positioned in the same direction as a conventional microsurgeon's forearms [11]. The body of the robot needs to be installed facing the telemicrosurgeon, as if the robot was about to perform a conventional microsurgical procedure. The telemicrosurgeon is comfortably seated at the master remote control console of the robot, distant from the patient. The telemicrosurgeon's forearms lie on the master console's armrests.

Adequate positioning of the robot is dictated by the anatomic area and required surgical exposure. In brachial plexus telemicrosurgery [12], the patient is placed in dorsal decubitus with a cushion under the scapula; the body of the robot is positioned at the back of the patient, between both the head and the shoulder undergoing surgery (Fig. 5.2a). In axillary nerve surgery [10], the patient is installed in lateral decubitus opposite to the nerve undergoing surgery; the body of the robot is positioned in front of the patient, next to the operated shoulder (Fig. 5.2b). In telemicrosurgery of the arm [6, 13], the patient is placed in dorsal decubitus, with 90° of abduction and 90° of external rotation of the shoulder and 90° of flexion in the elbow, on an armrest. The robot can be positioned on either sides of the trunk, with the body of the robot adjacent to the contralateral upper limb and the surgical instruments on the side of the upper limb undergoing surgery (Fig. 5.2c). In hand and forearm telemicrosurgery [5, 7], the patient is placed in dorsal decubitus. The shoulder is positioned on an armrest and abducted to 90°. The robot can be positioned on either sides of the arm with the body of the robot at the opposite side with regard to a conventional microsurgeon and with the instruments at the same side (Fig. 5.2d).

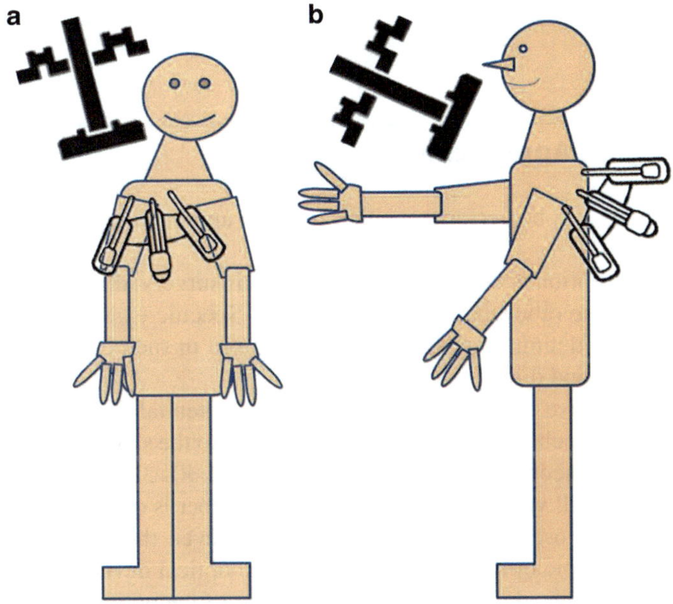

Fig. 5.2 Telemicrosurgical installations. (**a**) Brachial plexus. The body of the robot is positioned at the back of the patient, between both the head and the shoulder undergoing surgery. (**b**) Axillary nerve. The body of the robot is positioned in front of the patient. (**c**) Arm telemicrosurgery. The robot is positioned on both sides of the trunk, with the body of the robot on the side of the contralateral upper limb and the surgical instruments on the side of the upper limb undergoing surgery. (**d**) Hand and forearm telemicrosurgery. The robot is positioned on both sides of the arm with the body of the robot at the opposite side with regard to a conventional microsurgeon and with the instruments at the same side

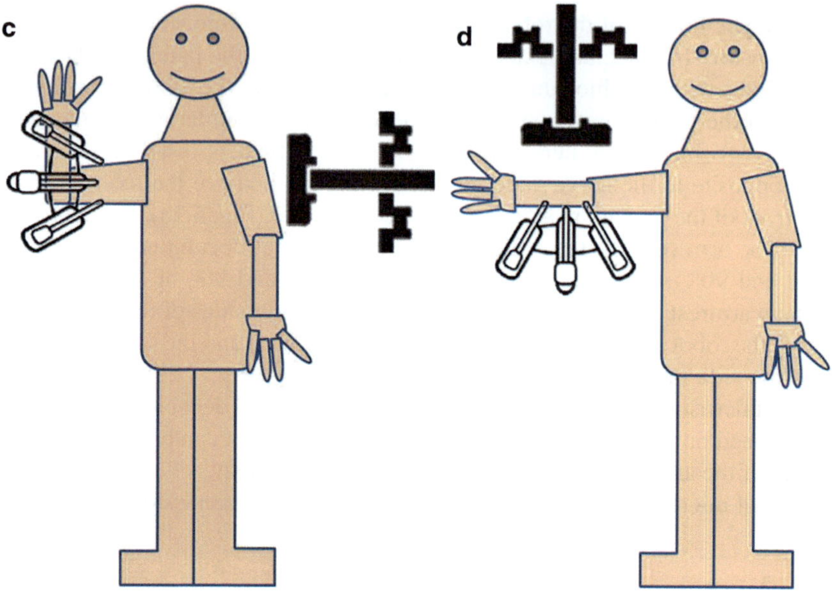

Fig. 5.2 (continued)

5.3 Surgical Approaches

Telemicrosurgery can be performed either by open approach or by minimally invasive means.

Using a conventional open approach, telemicrosurgery does not require any alteration in routine other than robot installation. Specific examples are described above. A 3D high-definition (HD), 0° camera is used in such cases as the surgical field view is large and direct.

Minimally invasive telemicrosurgery limits the potential for scar tissue formation. Surgical approaches and indications are subject to the same requirements as in conventional laparoscopic telesurgery [1]. An oblique 30° 3D HD optical device is used since the overall view inside the operating chamber is quite narrow. The same principles as in endoscopic surgery are employed, even though standard laparoscopic and endoscopic optical devices are 2D. The optical device has no degree of liberty inside the surgical chamber, and the rotation of the optical device around its axis provides a 360° vision. The three instrumental trocars and the optical trocar should all be separated by a minimum of 8 cm distance to avoid the arms of the robot coming into conflict. The four trocars should be inserted at least 8 cm deep into the surgical chamber to avoid extrusion from the cutaneous opening. The identifying mark on the body of the trocar represents the minimum depth of insertion and should be visible inside the surgical chamber. In addition, the portal width should not exceed 8 mm so as to prevent gas leaks in cases where CO_2 is used to maintain the chamber (Fig. 5.3a). Each trocar should be pushed inserted into the

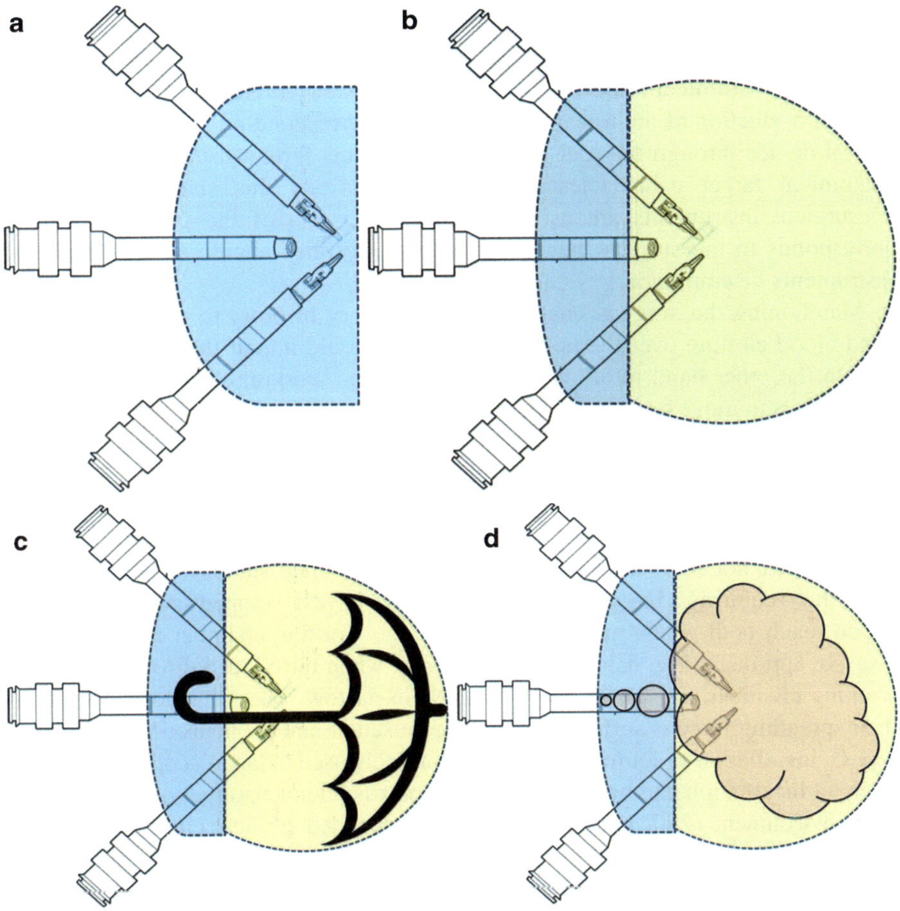

Fig. 5.3 Minimally invasive telemicrosurgical working chamber. (**a**) In *blue* is figured the working chamber into which the four trocars are introduced. (**b**) In *yellow* is figured the surgical field prolonging the working chamber. (**c**) Retractors spreading the planes of the working chamber. (**d**) Gas insufflation spreading the planes of the working chamber

cutaneous opening by means of a mandrel. It is much more reliable than a suture around the trocar to prevent both gas leaks and trocar extrusion.

5.4 Surgical Chamber

In telemicrosurgery, the surgical field is located inside a cavity which needs to be at first dissected and then maintained during the procedure.

Dissection of an adequate surgical chamber is obtained in two separate steps, according to a few precise rules. The first step consists of dissecting a subcutaneous space extending from each of the four surgical portals. This is performed by means of conventional forceps or scissors. When the four separate subcutaneous spaces rejoin so as to obtain a single space, the latter is then dissected as far as possible toward the anatomical target of the procedure (Fig. 5.3a). The second step consists of the introduction of the trocars along with the corresponding instruments and the optical device through the four portals. This permits further dissection toward the anatomical target using telesurgical instruments. At this stage, conventional telesurgical instruments are used. The deepest aspect of the surgical chamber corresponds to the surgical field (Fig. 5.3b). Only then should telemicrosurgical instruments be employed.

Maintaining the surgical chamber is compulsory in order to avoid on the one hand blood clotting over the optical lens which would impair the surgeon's vision and on the other hand to allow a sufficiently large working chamber for all four instruments to move smoothly. Two different methods are available: surgical retractors and gas insufflation. Both methods can be combined.

Retractors are routinely used in thyroid gland surgery through an axillary approach [9]. The axillary approach requires a several-centimeter scarring and a complementary mini-invasive thoracic approach for the third instrument. These retractors are not compatible with mini-invasive telemicrosurgery because they are rigid, thus requiring a large axillary approach. We have developed specific retractors which reach both goals: maintenance of a large working chamber and minimally invasive approach (Fig. 5.3c). These retractors, when introduced directly above the working chamber, are specifically indicated in narrow spaces inside the limbs, as their spreading force is sufficient regarding muscular and aponeurotic planes.

CO_2 insufflation at 4 mmHg pressure is routinely used in laparoscopic telesurgery. Such an insufflation can be used in brachial plexus telemicrosurgery, as a low-pressure environment is adequate to maintain an expanded surgical chamber, provided there are no leaks at the four minimally invasive trocar insertion points (Fig. 5.3d). Maximal pressure allowed in laparoscopic surgery is 15 mmHg [3, 8] in order to avoid subcutaneous emphysema [14]. This insufflation pressure is sufficient to maintain separation of limb muscular and aponeurotic planes during the surgical procedure.

Some authors propose a third method to help performance of endoscopic procedures at the limbs. Creation and maintenance of the dissection spaces is performed using inflatable balloons [15], but such devices require significant space and are therefore incompatible with telemicrosurgery since the latter requires anatomically targeted approaches extending several centimeters.

Conclusion

Installation of a telemicrosurgical procedure is complex, and adherence to several principles is warranted. The position of both the body and the arms of the robot should be thoroughly considered in order to access the surgical target at all time during the procedure. Correct positioning of the different minimally invasive surgical approaches is even more demanding to avoid any conflict between the arms of the robot. Dissection and maintenance of an adequate surgical working chamber is essential for free revolution of both the optical device and the instruments during the procedure. These rules will likely evolve in accordance with the further modifications of telemanipulators. Such modifications will likely occur in response to an expansion of telemicrosurgery applications to limb reconstructive procedures.

References

1. Ali MR, Rasmussen J, Bhasker Rao B (2007) Teaching robotic surgery: a stepwise approach. Surg Endosc 21:912–915
2. Chan W, Niranjan N, Ramakrishnan V (2010) Structured assessment of microsurgery skills in the clinical setting. J Plast Reconstr Aesthet Surg 63:1329–1334
3. Dexter SPL, Vucevic M, Gibson J, McMahon MJ (1999) Hemodynamic consequences of high- and low-pressure capnoperitoneum during laparoscopic cholecystectomy. Surg Endosc 13:376–381
4. Evans BC, Evans GR (2007) Microvascular surgery. Plast Reconstr Surg 119:18–30
5. Facca S, Liverneaux P (2010) Robotic assisted microsurgery in hypothenar hammer syndrome: a case report. Comput Aided Surg 15:110–114
6. Garcia JC Jr, Mantovani G, Gouzou S, Liverneaux P (2011) Telerobotic anterior translocation of the ulnar nerve. J Robotic Surg 5:153–156
7. Guldmann R, Pourtales MC, Liverneaux P (2010) Is it possible to use robots for carpal tunnel release? A case report. J Orthop Sci 15:430–433
8. Jacobs VR, Morrison JE Jr (2007) The real intraabdominal pressure during laparoscopy: comparison of different insufflators. J Minim Invasive Gynecol 14:103–107
9. Kang SW, Lee SC, Lee SH, Lee KY, Jeong JJ, Lee YS, Nam KH, Chang HS, Chung WY, Park CS (2007) Robotic thyroid surgery using a gasless, transaxillary approach and the da Vinci S system: the operative outcomes of 338 consecutive patients. Surgery 146:1048–1055
10. Lebailly F, Facca S, Bednar M, Mantovani G, Berner S, Liverneaux P (2010) Robotic surgery around shoulder girdle. In: Allieu Y (ed) Shoulder girdle. Sauramps Medical, Montpellier, pp 239–246
11. Liverneaux P, Nectoux E, Taleb C (2009) The future of robotics in hand surgery. Chir Main 28:278–285
12. Mantovani G, Liverneaux P, Berner S, Bednar M, Mohr C (2011) Endoscopic exploration and repair of brachial plexus with tele-robotic manipulation: a cadaver trial. J Neurosurg 8:1–6
13. Naito K, Facca S, Lequint T, Liverneaux P (2011) Oberlin's procedure for restoration of elbow flexion with Da Vinci robot: 4 cases. Plast Reconstruct Surg 129(3):707–711
14. Neuhaus SJ, Gupta A, Watson DI (2001) Helium and other alternative insufflation gases for laparoscopy. Surg Endosc 15:553–560
15. Zobrist R, Aponte RL, Levin LS (2002) Endoscopic access to the extremities: the principle of fascial clefts. J Orthop Trauma 16:264–271

Part II

Training

Earthworms

6

Gustavo Mantovani Ruggiero

6.1 Introduction

The training of microsurgery using the tele-manipulator surgical device does not differ in theory from conventional microsurgery [2].

After familiarizing oneself through the initial basic exercises, the trainee learns to manage the tele-manipulated arms, acquiring comfort with the 3D virtual image environment and triangulation. Training models include therapeutic toys for motor coordination training. The surgeon uses these inanimate training toys and the arms of the robot, moving rings along the wires, changing rings from different cones of rubber, and pinching and grasping different textures and materials (Fig. 6.1). During this step of training, the surgeon acquires the necessary skills requisite to operate the tele-manipulating equipment, including the joysticks, pedals, and several screen controls. Concurrently, the surgeon gains improved coordination of the movements of the robot arms and the control of the camera. It is also on those first steps of training that the basic information about the robotic system must be learned, including the external controls, equipment setup, and positioning over the surgical field.

Subsequently, procedure-specific training exercises may be undertaken. These exercises must try to simulate the different clinical situations presented on the diverse microsurgical procedures. The first training exercise on this stage is the simulation of a vessel anastomosis, manipulating artificial and biological tissue with tubular structure [2, 10].

Conventionally, at this point of training, the student usually starts using discarded biological materials such as human placenta or chicken wings before moving to the final stage of microvascular training using femoral arteries of living rats [1, 2].

G.M. Ruggiero, M.D.
Hand Surger Group, São Paulo Hand Center,
Beneficiencia Portuguesa de Sao Paulo Hospital,
Rua Maestro Cardim, 987, Sao Paolo 01323-001, Brazil
e-mail: mantovani@sphandcenter.com

P. Liverneaux et al. (eds.), *Telemicrosurgery*,
DOI 10.1007/978-2-8178-0391-3_6,

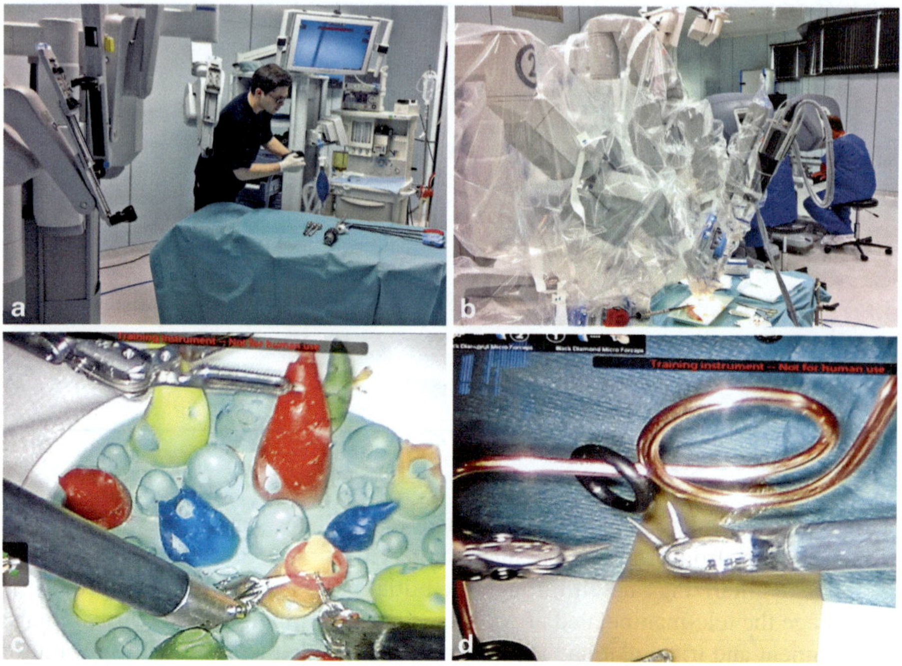

Fig. 6.1 Basic training on robotic microsurgery. (**a**) Instructor in action on the first steps of the robotic-microsurgery training. (**b**) Students practicing on second plane, the robot arms working on the first plane. (**c**) Rubber cones model for the first steps of training with the robot. (**d**) Bent wires with rings to basic training

6.2 Earthworms as a Training Model

The concept of using earthworms as an experimental model begun at Sao Paulo, Brazil, in 2005 in order to provide a substitute for human placenta or chicken parts, sometimes difficult to obtain for a training facility.

The first experience with the use of earthworms on conventional microsurgery training was successful and reported at literature on 2008 [4]. At the same year, this model was introduced to the research group of robotic microsurgery at Strasbourg University, France, and promptly adopted as one of the exercises on the first robotic microsurgery course (Fig. 6.2). This research on robotic microsurgery at Strasbourg University provided great advances on experimental surgery, including the feasibility and benefits of the robotics on nerves and small vessels procedures [3, 5, 8, 9].

After the inaugural course at Strasbourg, the earthworm model was used on a comparative research project performed at the same institution to evaluate the differences between robotic and conventional training, affirming its utility and simplicity [7]. In order to evaluate the success of the exercises, a patency test was described, consisting of catheterization of the earthworm segment after the suture and injection of saline fluid in one end, collecting the fluid at the other end and measuring the loss of fluid on the anastomosis site (Fig. 6.3).

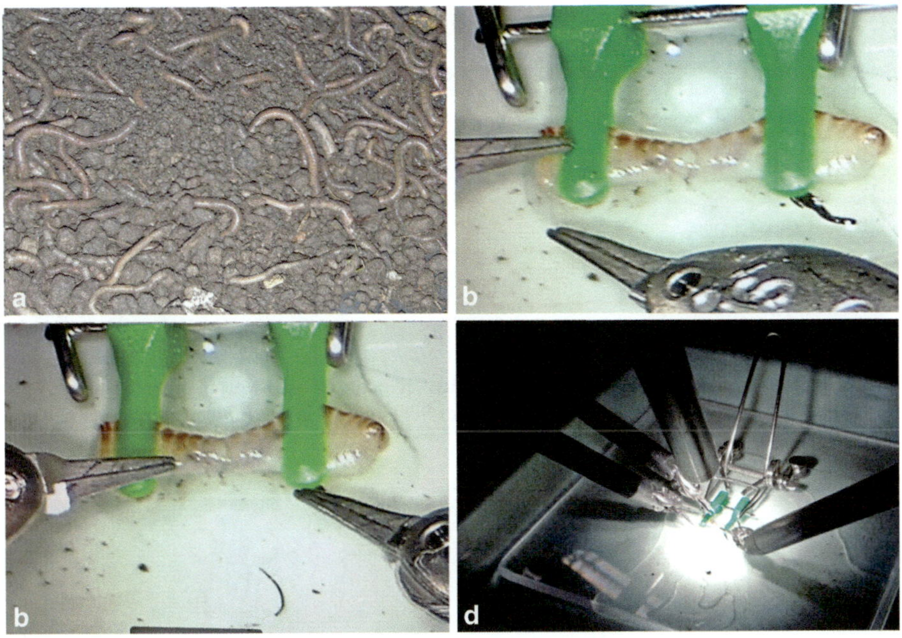

Fig. 6.2 Robotic microsurgery training with the earthworm model. (**a**) Source of earthworms. (**b**, **c**) Microscopic view of the exercise of end-to-end anastomosis with the da Vinci robot. (**d**) External view of the robot arms working on the earthworm exercise

6.3 Earthworms Used as a Model of Telemicrosurgey

The major benefits of this model are the minimal costs, the ease of preparation, and the worldwide availability. The earthworms can be obtained from the garden of the facility or acquired from a local humus producer. It is possible to obtain different sizes of earthworms with great variety of diameters. Each individual can provide enough material for at least three exercises since the preparation includes segmentation of the body in 1-in. pieces (Fig. 6.3a). The small pieces can be better handled and washed to remove the internal organs and provide, at the end of this process, a clean tubular body. This prepared segment can be then fixed with the traditional microvascular clamp stabilized on a small board and then manipulated by the robot. It is important to have a stable board with a fixation system to grab the clamp; otherwise, the clamp with the worm segment will be unsteady during the robot manipulation (Fig. 6.4b).

The exercise performed with this model is the simple end-to-end anastomosis (Fig. 6.2b, c) after simply sectioning the center of earthworm fixed on the clamp, but the lateral-end anastomosis can also be performed.

The muscular structure of the earthworm body provides an excellent simulation of the texture and fragility of a vascular structure (Fig. 6.4a), essential in the first steps of robotic training to recognize the "optic sensation" (ability to recognize the

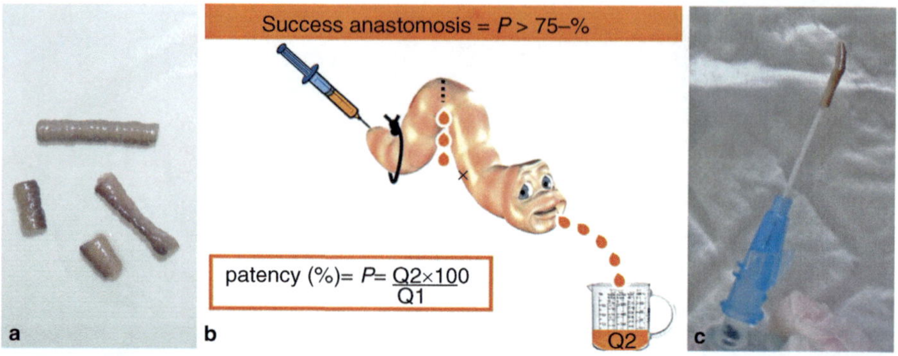

Fig. 6.3 Patency test using earthworm mode. (**a**) Segments of earthworms prepared to exercise. (**b**) Schematic explanation of the patency test. (**c**) Segment of earthworm catheterized to perform patency test

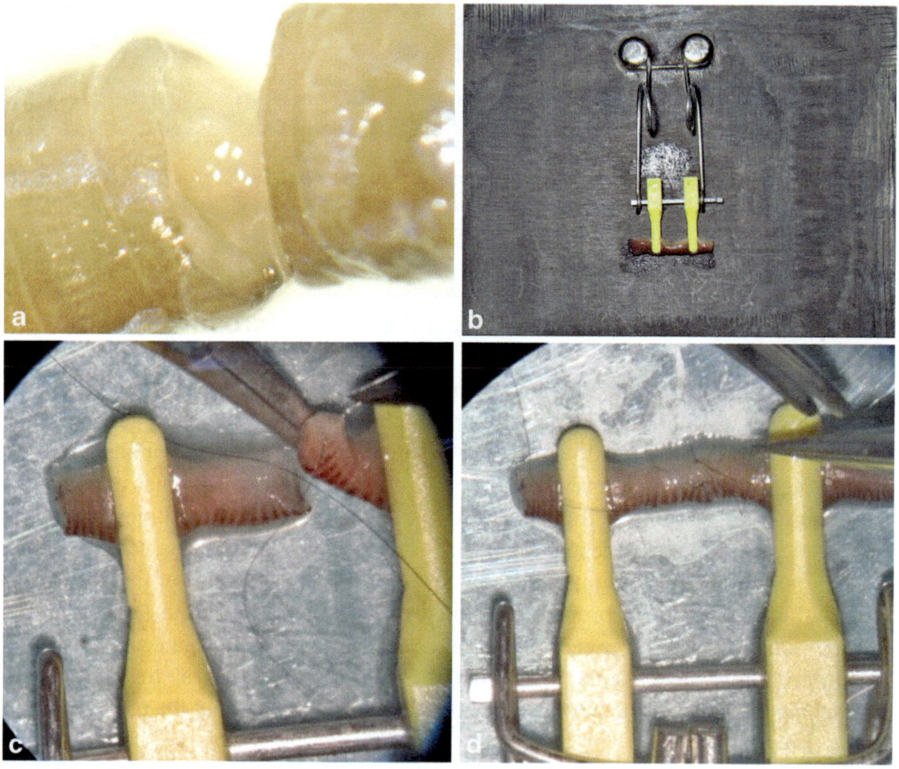

Fig. 6.4 Details of microsurgery training on earthworms. (**a**) Macro-view of the anastomosis site. (**b**) Metallic structure to stabilize the microvascular clamp during the exercise. (**c**, **d**) Microscopic view during earthworm suture to perform an end-to-end anastomosis

haptic sensation through the optic information). In truth, this represented one of the largest challenges in the beginnings of robotic microsurgery. There was doubt surrounding the ability of the surgeon to manipulate small and fragile suture threads such 9-0, 10-0, or 11-0 Nylon using a manipulated arms with absolutely no haptic feedback. Ultimately, this concern was laid to rest when the research using earthworms demonstrated that the tactile and haptic sensation was not necessary for these procedures, but only the optic feedback. In fact, a study made during the first training sessions confirmed that most the surgeons do not rely upon haptic feedback during conventional microsurgical procedures, since they are not able to feel the small variation of tension involved with fine caliber sutures, and the operator is primarily guided by optic feedback [6].

Conclusion

We recommend this model as a good alternative to an intermediate exercise between the artificial models exercises (latex gloves, silicon tubes) and the living animals models steps (rat femoral artery and vein). Finally, this situation provides the unexpected experience of having one of the most primitive creatures on earth manipulated by one of the highest technological advances of human medical sciences.

References

1. Hino A (2003) Training in microvascular surgery using a chicken wing artery. Neurosurgery 52:1495–1497; discussion 1497–1498
2. Kim J, Shaw Wilgis EF, Fanua SP (2001) Alternative model for teaching microsurgery. Microsurgery 21:379–382
3. Liverneaux P, Nectoux E, Taleb C (2009) The future of robotics in hand surgery. Chir Main 28:278–285
4. Mantovani G, Fukushima WY, Baik Cho A, Aita MA, Mazzetti MV (2009) Use of earthworms for microsurgery training. J Reconstr Microsurg 25:275–278
5. Nectoux E, Taleb C, Liverneaux P (2009) Nerve repair in telemicrosurgery: an experimental study. J Reconstr Microsurg 25:261–265
6. Panchulidze I, Berner S, Mantovani G, Liverneaux P (2011) Is haptic feedback necessary to microsurgical suturing? Comparative study of 9/0 and 10/0 knot tying operated by 24 surgeons. Hand Surg 16:1–3
7. Ramdhian R, Bednar M, Mantovani G, Facca S, Liverneaux P (2011) Microsurgery and telemicrosurgery training: a comparative study. J Reconstr Microsurg 27(9):537–542
8. Taleb C, Nectoux E, Liverneaux PA (2008) Telemicrosurgery: a feasibility study in a rat model. Chir Main 27:104–108
9. Taleb C, Nectoux E, Liverneaux P (2009) Limb replantation with two robots: a feasibility study in a pig model. Microsurgery 29:232–235
10. Usón J, Calles MC (2002) Design of a new suture practice card for microsurgical training. Microsurgery 22:324–328

Vessels 7

Joo-Yup Lee and Alexander Y. Shin

7.1 Introduction

Since the introduction of operating microscope and precision instruments, microsurgery has been evolved significantly for several decades [25]. The full potential of microsurgery, however, is limited by the individual surgeon's precision and manual dexterity. For example, there is no interface to filter physiological tremor between surgeons' hands and their microsurgical instrument. Moreover, movements are limited by the physiological articular amplitude of their wrists.

The development of robotic surgical systems to assist surgeons in performing microsurgery may be the answer to overcome the surgical limitations imposed by the precision motions and physical demands of microsurgery. By digitizing the surgeon's movements, this system has the potential to remove surgical tremor and scale surgical movements to facilitate fine motor dexterity [6]. As microsurgery often takes human dexterity to the limit, it is important for microsurgeons to pay attention to the robotic surgical systems in particular the ability to advance the science and art of microsurgery. The feasibility of carrying out different microsurgical procedures with robotic systems has been well documented [10, 11, 13, 16, 23, 24].

The use of this new technology has raised several important issues regarding surgical education and training. The robotic interface is different to microvascular anastomosis under the operating microscope because it involves remote surgical control, stereoscopic vision, and lack of haptic feedback. In order to avoid problems

J. Lee, M.D., Ph.D.
Department of Orthopedic Surgery, The Catholic University of Korea, Seoul, Korea

A.Y. Shin, M.D. (✉)
Department of Orthopedic Surgery, Mayo Clinic, 200 1st Street SW, Rochester, MN 55905, USA
e-mail: shin.alexander@mayo.edu

P. Liverneaux et al. (eds.), *Telemicrosurgery*,
DOI 10.1007/978-2-8178-0391-3_7, © Springer-Verlag France 2013

that could occur with robotic-assisted microsurgery in the clinical setting, appropriate training, development of skills, and assessment of outcomes need to be established in a laboratory/teaching setting.

This chapter will review the current training in conventional microsurgery and the methods for assessing surgical skill training. We will also discuss the important parameters in the learning curve of microvascular anastomosis and the future direction of training for robotic-assisted microvascular anastomosis.

7.2 Current Methods of Training in Microsurgery

Microsurgery is a complex procedure and requires significant amount of training. There are several reasons that microsurgical procedures are demanding. First, the microscope magnifies and exaggerates all movements, while it limits visual field and depth. Second, microsurgery requires that the surgeon spend long hours in the same relatively fixed posture. This immobility can be physically demanding and taxing during long, complex procedures and can adversely affect the surgeon's technical performance. Third, physiological tremor is magnified in proportion to the length of the instrument and so reduces precision and dexterity. Because of these obstacles and complexity of the procedures, microsurgical competence cannot be acquired by observation or by performing them infrequently. It also requires continual training or participation in microsurgical procedures to prevent loss of the dexterity and stamina.

Traditional methods of surgical training have been done in the operating room under the supervision of senior surgeons [20]. However, it has been recognized that this method needs to be revised with current changes in healthcare system (reduction in working hours, pressures on operating room efficiency, and the ethical consideration of training on patients) [2]. Nowadays, attending microsurgical skill training courses has become an increasingly popular method of practical skill acquisition. These courses usually run over several consecutive days teaching microsurgery technique using simulators or animals in the laboratory setting [12]. The efficacy of the microsurgical training course was proved in several studies [1, 4]. Atkins et al. [1] found that attendance at the microsurgical training course resulted in an improvement in microsurgical skills in a majority of trainees. However, attending a course does not guarantee that an individual has reached competent operative ability. It is crucial for microsurgical trainees to continuously develop highly refined manual dexterity, hand-eye coordination, and sound clinical judgment. Technical skills, knowledge, as well as dexterity play a major role in microsurgical competence [4].

7.3 Assessment of Training

Currently there are five methods of assessment in surgery used to assess technical skills, and all vary in the degree of reliability and validity (Table 7.1) [19]. Procedure lists with logs without any description of the quality of the performance are

Table 7.1 Technical skills assessment: available approaches

Method	Reliability	Validity
Procedure lists with logs	N/A	Poor
Direct observation	Poor	Modest
Direct observation with criteria	High	High
Animal models with criteria	High	Proportional to realism
Videotapes	High	Proportional to realism

a conventional method of assessment and are useful to record the progress and completion of a surgical training. However, construct validity is poor since it does not relate to the surgeon's level of skill and surgical competence [5]. Additionally, procedure logs do not guarantee that the procedures have been done well.

Direct observing trainees performing surgical procedure is mostly subjective and lacks reliability and construct validity. Although an experienced surgeon might be capable of making a judgment of technical performances, this method is usually unreliable unless the judgment is made with specific predetermined criteria.

To directly and objectively measure surgical training, new tools to assess surgical dexterity have been developed. One such validated method is global rating scale of objective structured assessment of technical skill (OSATS) (Table 7.2) [14]. The OSATS score includes several parameters to assess surgical performance. Each parameter is scored from one to five and then a global score is calculated. This score has been modified and used in various surgical fields [17, 21, 22, 26]. It is also used in training of conventional microsurgery as well [1]. If preceptors were trained to use the assessment forms, evidence showed that OSATS score had consistently found to be valid and reliable [14].

A disadvantage of this type of assessment is that the preceptor must be present throughout the procedure. Video recordings can be used to overcome this drawback as it can be done at a convenient time, but it remains time consuming and expensive.

7.4 Learning Curve

The learning curve can be defined as an improvement in performance with experience and practice [18]. This improvement tends to be more rapid at first and then decreases over time as the curve reaches a plateau. This term is being used increasingly to denote this phenomenon of gaining knowledge and improving skills in performing a surgical procedure. In learning curve, three main features can be recognized. An initial or starting level defines where the performance level begins. The learning rate measures how quickly a particular level of performance is reached. Last, the asymptote or learning plateau is the level at which performance stabilized (Fig. 7.1). Although learning curves have been observed for many health technologies including robotic-assisted surgery and described by dividing the data arbitrarily, they are rarely quantified by statistical analysis [18]. Another problem in studying

Table 7.2 Global rating scale of objective structured assessment of technical skills (OSATS)

Respect for tissue	1	2	3	4	5
	Frequently used unnecessary force on tissue or caused damage by inappropriate use of instruments		Careful handling of tissue but occasionally caused inadvertent damage		Consistently handled tissues appropriately with minimal tissue damage, no rough handling
Time and motion	1	2	3	4	5
	Many unnecessary moves		Efficient time/motion but some unnecessary moves		Clear economy of movement and maximum efficiency
Instrument handling	1	2	3	4	5
	Repeatedly makes tentative or awkward moves with instruments		Competent use of instruments although occasionally appeared stiff or awkward		Fluid moves with instruments and no awkwardness
Knowledge of instruments	1	2	3	4	5
	Frequently asked for the wrong instrument or used an inappropriate instrument		Knew names of most instruments and used appropriate instrument		Obviously familiar with the instruments required and their names
Flow of operation	1	2	3	4	5
	Frequently stopped operating and seemed unsure of next move		Demonstrated some forward planning with reasonable progression of procedure		Obviously planned course of operation with effortless flow from one move to the next
Knowledge of specific procedure	1	2	3	4	5
	Deficient knowledge. Needed specific instruction at most steps		Knew all important steps of operation		Demonstrated familiarity with all aspects of operation
Quality of anastomosis	1	2	3	4	5
	Crossed and tangled suture material, sloppy knots, imprecise inconsistent suture placement		Minimal tangling, mostly square knots, good suture placement and consistency with some variability		Excellent suture material control, square knots, short clean knot tails, precise, consistent suture placement

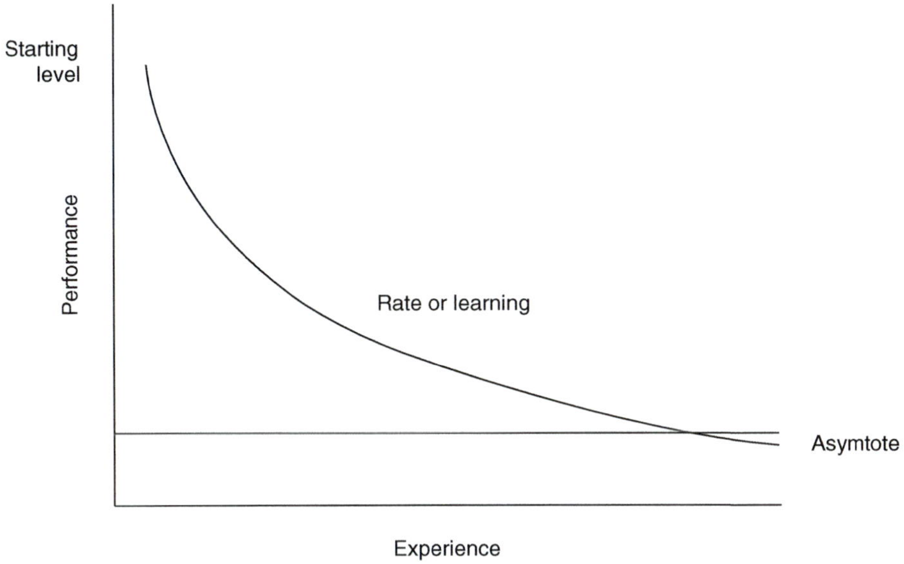

Fig. 7.1 Parameters of the learning curve

learning curve is the identification of reliable measures of learning. Many studies have used complications or conversions as the proxies for learning, which might be relatively infrequent or unreliable [3]. Other proxies for learning, such as duration of an operation, were also used because it is easy to analyze statistically. As operation time alone does not necessarily indicate better performance, assessment should be used in context with other methods of assessment such as OSATS score.

Recently, we studied the learning effect of robotic-assisted microvascular anastomosis in a rat model and hypothesized that the learning rate as well as the learning plateau of robotic-assisted microvascular anastomosis could be estimated precisely using curve fitting technique. Three surgeons with various microsurgical experiences performed 20 microsurgical anastomosis of the rat femoral artery using da Vinci robotic system (Intuitive surgical, Inc., Sunnyvale, CA, USA). We evaluated anastomosis time, patency rate, and quality of anastomosis. OSATS score which is introduced to assess surgical dexterity was also measured. Using a nonlinear regression model, an inverse power law curve ($Y=a+b*X^{-c}$) was fit for each surgeon's anastomosis time and OSATS score, yielding an estimate of the learning rate and the learning plateau (Figs. 7.2 and 7.3).

In this study, we found important aspects of learning curve including the learning plateau, and the learning rate could be estimated by curve fitting technique. We also found that the patency rate correlated with OSATS score and quality of anastomosis rather than anastomosis time (unpublished data). As anastomosis time does not necessarily correlate with the patency rate, OSATS score might be a valuable tool to evaluate trainees during robotic-assisted microvascular anastomosis training.

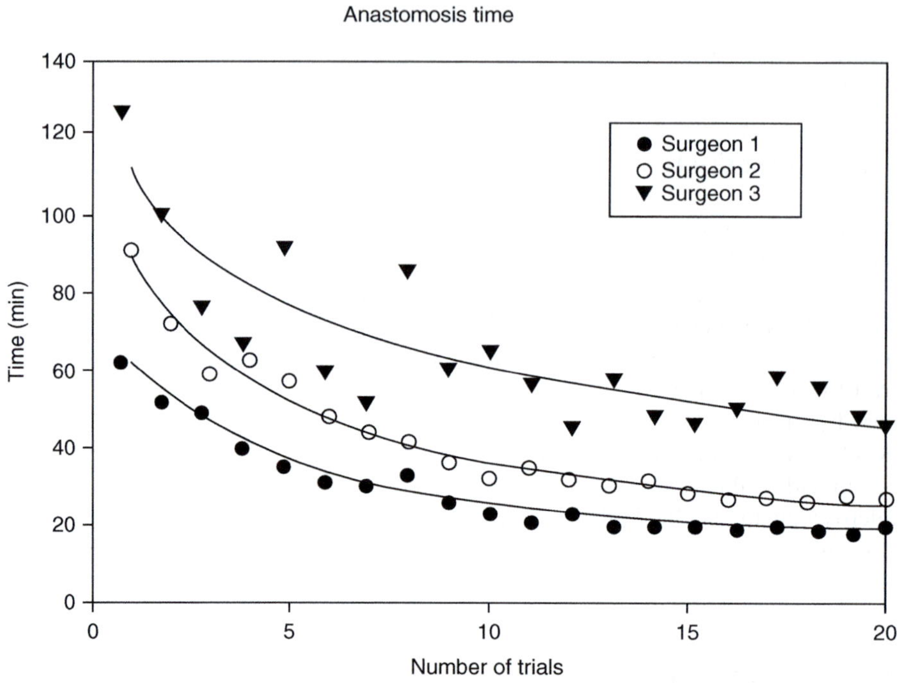

Fig. 7.2 Learning curves of anastomosis time during robotic-assisted microvascular anastomosis performed by three surgeons with different microsurgical experiences

7.5 Training in Robotic-Assisted Microsurgery

It is unknown whether prior conventional microsurgical experience is required to develop competence in robotic-assisted microsurgery. In the field of general surgery, there have been studies to assess the issues about transfer of training in robotic-assisted surgery. De Ugarte et al. [7] observed that the residents who practiced with the robot first did no better than those who started with conventional instruments suggests that the conventional surgical skills were not transferable to a robotic model. Figert et al. [8] postulated that no transfer of training occurs from open surgical experience to laparoscopic surgery because laparoscopy presents a completely new set of skills that must be learned. In one study about transfer of training in robotic-assisted microsurgery, Karamanoukian et al. [9] concluded that robotic-assisted microvascular anastomosis can be mastered equally well by surgical trainees and fully trained vascular surgeons. In fact, the motions required to manipulate the robot are distinct from those required for conventional instruments. The added benefit of articulation may in fact impair learning of conventional techniques by "spoiling" trainees who become accustomed to it [7]. For this reason, we recommend that trainees practice with conventional instruments first before training with the robot.

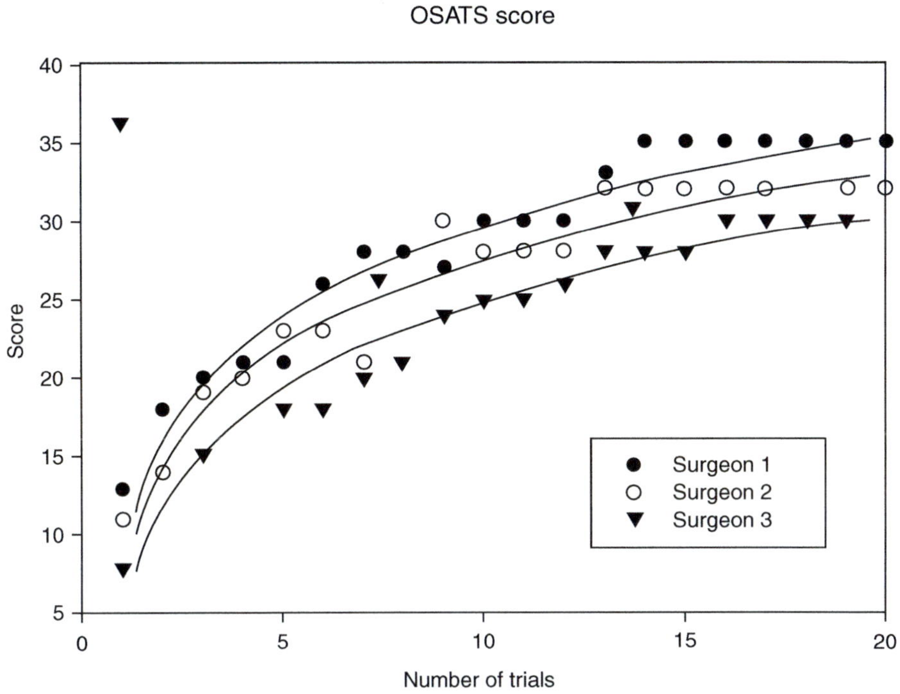

Fig. 7.3 Learning curves of OSATS score during robotic-assisted microvascular anastomosis performed by three surgeons with different microsurgical experiences

With the growth of robotic-assisted surgery in the field of general surgery and urology, legal and ethical issues in training and credentialing robotic surgery have risen [15, 27]. A potential medicolegal implication arises for the preceptor in the event of malpractice by the trainee. Unfortunately there is no standardized training and credentialing system to evaluate surgeon competency in general surgery and urology. While preceptors have a crucial role in observing and certifying surgeon competence, the need for a governing body to establish the standards for a surgeon to become a preceptor cannot be overemphasized. Currently the robotic company (Intuitive surgical, Inc., Sunnyvale, CA, USA) requires a minimum of 20 completed robotic cases to become a preceptor. The skill level of preceptors might be heterogenous, and it is far from ideal for ensuring trainee competency.

The Society of Urologic Robotic Surgeons recently suggested recommendations for the safe implementation and credentialing of robotic-assisted radical prostatectomy at an institution [27]. They suggested that the central certification authority, rather than the robotic industry, should assume responsibility for identifying and promoting expert robotic surgeons. We are in general agreement with their suggestion. As established microsurgeons at our respective institutions, we have had significant experience running regional or institutional microsurgery training courses. If robotic-assisted microsurgery becomes clinical reality, this experience might be extended to establish robotic microsurgery training center in the near future.

Conclusions

The primary benefits of the robot are the elimination of tremor, the ability to downscale motion, the extra degree of motion, and the ergonomic position of the surgeon. Although the roles and applications of robotic-assisted microsurgery are yet to be defined, it is promising to have a revolutionary future in the field of microsurgery.

Training and assessment for robotic-assisted microsurgery is a complex procedure, and these need to be accompanied by constructive feedback from experienced microsurgeons. The guidelines and recommendations for preceptoring robotic-assisted microsurgery will be necessary to ensure the safety of patients and surgeons while initiating a robotic microsurgery program at an individual institution.

References

1. Atkins JL, Kalu PU, Lannon DA et al (2005) Training in microsurgical skills: does course-based learning deliver? Microsurgery 25:481–485
2. Balasundaram I, Aggarwal R, Darzi LA (2010) Development of a training curriculum for microsurgery. Br J Oral Maxillofac Surg 48:598–606
3. Bull C, Yates R, Sarkar D et al (2000) Scientific, ethical, and logistical considerations in introducing a new operation: a retrospective cohort study from paediatric cardiac surgery. BMJ 320:1168–1173
4. Chan WY, Matteucci P, Southern SJ (2007) Validation of microsurgical models in microsurgery training and competence: a review. Microsurgery 27:494–499
5. Cuschieri A, Francis N, Crosby J et al (2001) What do master surgeons think of surgical competence and revalidation? Am J Surg 182:110–116
6. Damiano RJ Jr, Reichenspurner H, Ducko CT (2000) Robotically assisted endoscopic coronary artery bypass grafting: current state of the art. Adv Card Surg 12:37–57
7. De Ugarte DA, Etzioni DA, Gracia C et al (2003) Robotic surgery and resident training. Surg Endosc 17:960–963
8. Figert PL, Park AE, Witzke DB et al (2001) Transfer of training in acquiring laparoscopic skills. J Am Coll Surg 193:533–537
9. Karamanoukian RL, Bui T, McConnell MP et al (2006) Transfer of training in robotic-assisted microvascular surgery. Ann Plast Surg 57:662–665
10. Karamanoukian RL, Finley DS, Evans GR et al (2006) Feasibility of robotic-assisted microvascular anastomoses in plastic surgery. J Reconstr Microsurg 22:429–431
11. Katz RD, Rosson GD, Taylor JA et al (2005) Robotics in microsurgery: use of a surgical robot to perform a free flap in a pig. Microsurgery 25:566–569
12. Klein I, Steger U, Timmermann W et al (2003) Microsurgical training course for clinicians and scientists at a German University hospital: a 10-year experience. Microsurgery 23:461–465
13. Le Roux PD, Das H, Esquenazi S et al (2001) Robot-assisted microsurgery: a feasibility study in the rat. Neurosurgery 48:584–589
14. Martin JA, Regehr G, Reznick R et al (1997) Objective structured assessment of technical skill (OSATS) for surgical residents. Br J Surg 84:273–278

15. Mavroforou A, Michalodimitrakis E, Hatzitheo-Filou C et al (2010) Legal and ethical issues in robotic surgery. Int Angiol 29:75–79
16. Nectoux E, Taleb C, Liverneaux P (2009) Nerve repair in telemicrosurgery: an experimental study. J Reconstr Microsurg 25:261–265
17. Nielsen PE, Foglia LM, Mandel LS et al (2003) Objective structured assessment of technical skills for episiotomy repair. Am J Obstet Gynecol 189:1257–1260
18. Ramsay CR, Grant AM, Wallace SA et al (2001) Statistical assessment of the learning curves of health technologies. Health Technol Assess 5:1–79
19. Reznick RK (1993) Teaching and testing technical skills. Am J Surg 165:358–361
20. Rutkow IM (1978) William Stewart Halsted and the Germanic influence on education and training programs in surgery. Surg Gynecol Obstet 147:602–606
21. Siddiqui NY, Stepp KJ, Lasch SJ et al (2008) Objective structured assessment of technical skills for repair of fourth-degree perineal lacerations. Am J Obstet Gynecol 199:671–676
22. Swift SE, Carter JF (2006) Institution and validation of an observed structured assessment of technical skills (OSATS) for obstetrics and gynecology residents and faculty. Am J Obstet Gynecol 195:617–621; discussion 621–613
23. Taleb C, Nectoux E, Liverneaux PA (2008) Telemicrosurgery: a feasibility study in a rat model. Chir Main 27:104–108
24. Taleb C, Nectoux E, Liverneaux P (2009) Limb replantation with two robots: a feasibility study in a pig model. Microsurgery 29:232–235
25. Tamai S (2009) History of microsurgery. Plast Reconstr Surg 124:e282–e294
26. VanBlaricom AL, Goff BA, Chinn M et al (2005) A new curriculum for hysteroscopy training as demonstrated by an objective structured assessment of technical skills (OSATS). Am J Obstet Gynecol 193:1856–1865
27. Zorn KC, Gautam G, Shalhav AL et al (2009) Training, credentialing, proctoring and medicolegal risks of robotic urological surgery: recommendations of the society of urologic robotic surgeons. J Urol 182:1126–1132

Nerves

8

Stacey H. Berner

8.1 Introduction

Neural tissue is among the most difficult tissues to operate on, since it requires mastership of microsurgical techniques prior to acquiring robotic skills. This may represent a real triumph of telemanipulators, as they facilitate the microsurgical step. Among the other assets developed, the two most important ones are the suppression of physiological tremor and the gearing down of movements up to six times, enhancing overall gesture precision [4]. Robotic training protocols have been developed and continue to develop. The goals of the training programs are to build facility with the robot and to provide an opportunity to simulate an in vivo or "live" surgical procedure. Familiarity with the instrumentation and practice with the telemanipulator are vital to successful completion of training in robotic nerve repair. Various exercises have been developed which require the surgeon to use two instruments simultaneously to manipulate synthetic materials (Fig. 8.1). These exercises are designed to train the surgeon to become facile in moving the camera in the x-, y-, and z-axes (medial-lateral, up-down, in-out). Adjustments of the operative field of view with the da Vinci robot can easily be performed with the camera pedal. Once the surgeon has gained a comfort level in adjusting field of view, it is time to become more familiar with the instruments.

Refinements in instrumentation are ongoing, but presently, the Black Diamond forceps (Intuitive Surgical, Sunnyvale, CA, USA) are the preferred instrument attachments for microneural repair using the da Vinci Robot. Avoidance of grasping the suture needle simultaneously with each Black Diamond forceps will help preserve needle integrity. To facilitate seamless completion of an anastomosis, use of a Potts scissors in the 3rd robotic arm can be helpful for dissection and cutting sutures.

S.H. Berner, M.D.
Department of Orthopedic Surgery, Northwest Hospital,
10 Crossroads Drive, Suite 210, Owings Mills, Baltimore, MD, USA
e-mail: sberner@surgcenter.com

P. Liverneaux et al. (eds.), *Telemicrosurgery*,
DOI 10.1007/978-2-8178-0391-3_8, © Springer-Verlag France 2013

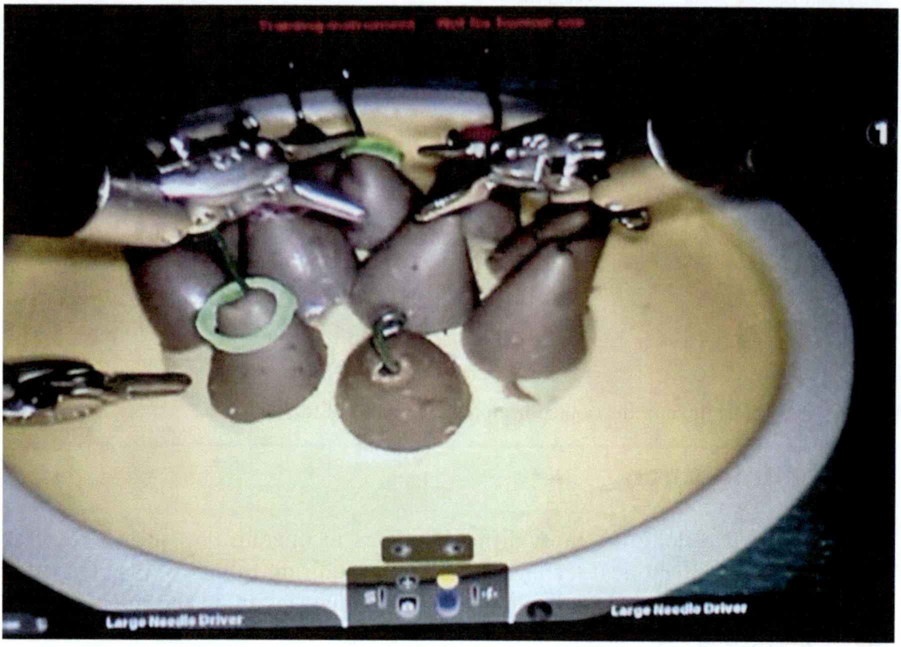

Fig. 8.1 Synthetic training apparatus

Once the surgeon is comfortable utilizing the instruments to manipulate fine suture and needles, he or she can progress to experimental nerve repair.

8.2 Robot-Assisted Nerve Repair Model

There are various experimental approaches that can be utilized to improve overall dexterity and improve precision. For those surgeons who are interested in mastering a particular surgical maneuver or technique, procedure-specific models have been developed. For those models to be successful, they need to accurately simulate the in vivo surgical environment. For certain structures, such as skin, the tissue properties have been adequately represented with synthetic materials. However, to date, there is not an adequate synthetic substitute or training model for nerve surgery and microneural repair. As such, the surgeon interested in learning the skill of robot-assisted nerve repair requires training on animal and cadaver tissue. The sciatic nerve of a rat is an excellent structure for simulating in vivo microneural repair (Fig. 8.2).

Robotic training for nerve surgery and nerve repair requires access to a training center with advanced capabilities. Nerve decompression surgery has been performed using the da Vinci Robot [2, 3]. To perform nerve decompression, one needs to have a clear understanding of the anatomic relationships in the environment of the nerve. Our understanding of three-dimensional anatomy will likely

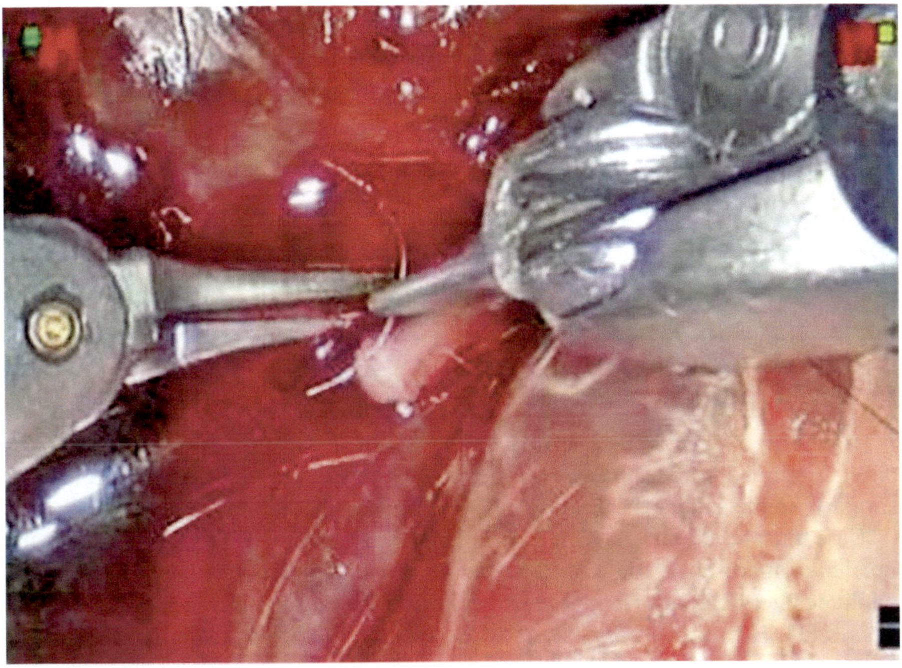

Fig. 8.2 Repair of sciatic nerve of rat with 10/0 nylon suture (Courtesy of Philippe Liverneaux)

evolve as robotic-assisted nerve surgery becomes more commonplace. The surgeon may not be accustomed to viewing the extra-articular constituents of the musculoskeletal system using endoscopy or when viewing in a narrow field. This latter circumstance is similar to using an operative microscope. Hence, orientation is critical to success and to avoidance of complications. Once this appreciation of the anatomic relationships is gained, the ability to perform nerve decompression surgery, neurolysis, or even neurectomy is predicated on the ability to maneuver and manipulate the robotic arms and specialized attachments. Soft tissue dissection is a relatively straightforward skill to master. The use of cadaver materials aids in gaining familiarity with the anatomy as seen through the stereoscopic viewer of the robot. It is of additional great benefit to perform a confirmatory open dissection after completing the robotically assisted nerve decompression, neurolysis, or neurectomy. Clinical applications may include neurolysis of the brachial plexus, nerve decompression in the upper or lower extremity, neurectomy for treatment of spasticity, and translocation of neuromata.

Advanced robotic training may utilize the endoscopic capabilities of the telemanipulator to perform minimally invasive nerve repair. This has been demonstrated in an experimental endoscopic repair of a brachial plexus lesion [5] (Fig. 8.3a, b).

Robotic nerve repair is associated with many of the same challenges as conventional repair with an operating microscope. Adequate magnification can be provided with each methodology. Currently, magnification up to 10x can be achieved with the

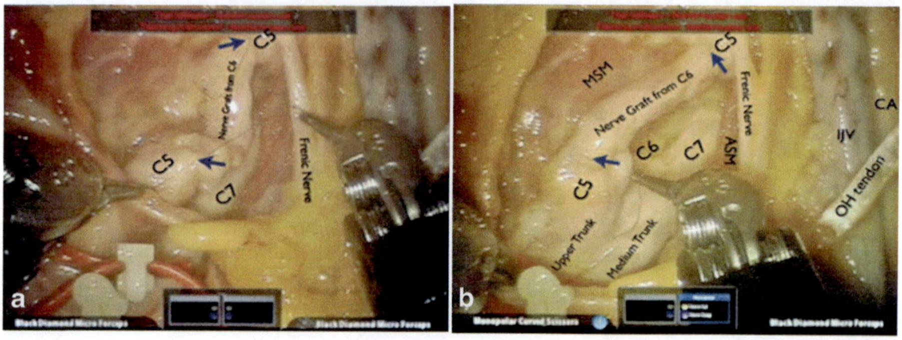

Fig. 8.3 (**a**) Experimental lesion brachial plexus. (**b**) Repair with nerve graft, C6-C5

da Vinci surgical robot (Intuitive Surgical Inc, Sunnyvale, CA, USA). This compares similarly to the standard operating microscope magnification.

Care must be exercised when utilizing fine suture material. Proponents of use the operative microscope for traditional nerve repair suggest that haptical feedback facilitates nerve repair. Haptical feedback is the perception of pressures applied to tissues [1]. However, in a study of 24 experienced surgeons using 9/0- and 10/0-knot-tying technique with handheld micro-forceps and needle holders, haptical feedback was not noted to be associated with the surgeon's ability to adequately tie knots and maintain suture integrity. Visualization likely is the critical component for adequate suture and knot management when performing microneural repair with fine suture materials [6].

Comparison of conventional microsurgery with telemicrosurgery tends to show comparable results in terms of repair quality, a shorter operating time with conventional microsurgery, and an incredibly improved comfort in ergonomics with telemanipulators [4]. Operating time will likely be reduced as specialized microsurgical instruments are developed. An additional potential benefit that telemanipulators present with that conventional microsurgery lacks is the possibility to work simultaneously with two robots; thanks to the very small steric hindrance in the operating field [7]. Both operators by means of their telemanipulator can perform a portion of a complex, nervous microsurgical repair, thus gaining on operating time. In conventional microsurgery, steric hindrance of the hands and the forearms of a surgeon make it impossible for two surgeons to work on a difficult procedure at the same time.

Conclusion

The interested and committed surgeon can master the requisite skills to perform nerve decompression, neuroma resection, neurectomy, and nerve repair with the aid of a robotic telemanipulator. Once facility has been achieved in the lab, transition to the clinical setting can be rewarding. Training protocols will continue to evolve and become standardized as this emerging discipline grows.

References

1. Cotin S, Delingette H, Ayache N (2000) A hybrid elastic model allowing realtime cutting, deformation and force-feedback for surgery training and simulation. Vis Comp J 16:437–452
2. Garcia JC Jr, Mantovani G, Gouzou S et al (2011) Telerobotic anterior translocation of the ulnar nerve. J Robot Surg 5:153–156
3. Guldmann R, Pourtales MC, Liverneaux P (2010) Is it possible to use robots for carpal tunnel release? J Orthop Sci 15:430–433
4. Liverneaux P, Nectoux E, Taleb C (2009) The future of robotics in hand surgery. Chir Main 28:278–285
5. Mantovani G, Liverneaux P, Garcia JC et al (2011) Endoscopic exploration and repair of brachial plexus with tele-robotic manipulation: a cadaver trial. J Neurosurg 8:1–6
6. Panchulidze I, Berner S, Mantovani G et al (2011) Is haptic feedback necessary to microsurgical suturing? A comparative study of 9/0 and 10/0knot tying operated by 24 surgeons. Hand Surg 16:1–3
7. Taleb C, Nectoux E, Liverneaux P (2009) Limb replantation with two robots: a feasibility study in a pig model. Microsurgery 29:232–235

Part III

Experimental Research

9 Free Tissue Transfer

Stacey H. Berner

9.1 Introduction

In free tissue transfer, a segment of skin, fascia, muscle, tendon, bone, or a composite of any or all of these structures is isolated on its vascular pedicle. The donor tissue is then separated from its indigenous location and attached to a recipient site. Anastomosis of the donor inflow artery and outflow vein to the local blood supply is performed, immediately restoring the viability of the donor tissue. Free tissue transfer usually requires magnification and is therefore classified as a microsurgical procedure.

Microvascular anastomosis of small caliber blood vessels was initially described in 1960 by Jacobson and Suarez [6]. This represents the first usage of the term "microsurgery." Chen et al. reported on a successful arm replantation in 1963 in the *Chinese Medical Journal* [2]. Kleinert et al. issued the first report of microsurgical repair of digital vessels in 1963 [7]. Nakayama, a Japanese cardiothoracic surgeon, reported the first true series of microsurgical free tissue transfers using vascularized intestinal segments to the neck for esophageal reconstruction after cancer resections using 3–4 mm vessels [9]. Thus, the modern era of free tissue transfer was born.

During the late 1960s and early 1970s, there was significant growth in the field of reconstructive microsurgery. The first human microsurgical transplantation of the second toe-to-thumb likely occurred in February 1966 by Dr. Dong-yue Yang and Yu-dong Gu, in Shanghai China as noted in the report of the American Transplant Mission [1]. The first published report of great toe-to-thumb transfer was performed in April 1968 by Mr. John Cobbett, in England [3].Throughout the remainder of the decade of the 1970s, an expansion in the number of free tissue transfers is noted in the literature [5, 8]. As greater knowledge of the axial pattern of blood vessel territories was gained, an increase in the variety of donor flaps was noted [5, 8].

S.H. Berner, M.D.
Department of Orthopedic Surgery, Northwest Hospital,
10 Crossroads Drive, Suite 210, Owings Mills, Baltimore, MD, USA
e-mail: sberner@surgcenter.com

P. Liverneaux et al. (eds.), *Telemicrosurgery*,
DOI 10.1007/978-2-8178-0391-3_9, © Springer-Verlag France 2013

The donor material can include soft tissue elements, bone, or both. The donor material can be of autogenous or allogenic nature. Autogenous donor tissue should not leave the host with a greater functional deficit than that which is gained through the tissue transfer process. This requirement does not necessarily apply to allogenic transfers or transplants.

9.2 Robot-Assisted Free Tissue Transfer Models

Improvements in magnification devices and optics have enhanced the surgeon's ability to perform successful free tissue transfer. Surgeon training and experience lead to greater precision. Precision becomes a critical determinant of viability of the transferred part when surgeons attempt to transfer smaller and more delicate tissues. As such, use of a tele-manipulator holds great promise for the fields of transplantation and tissue transfer. Robotic telemanipulators increase surgical precision through the demultiplication effect. Physiological tremor is a well-known phenomenon in conventional microsurgery. Telesurgery allows suppression of this tremor by gearing down operative gesture [4]. Surgical telemanipulator robotic devices may additionally benefit the surgeon by decreasing fatigue. Hand and clutch mechanisms can be immediately activated if the surgeon finds himself in an awkward or perilous position when dealing with delicate or critical structures. This allows a brief rest and subsequent repositioning of the surgeon's hands and the animated instruments so as to avoid tissue damage in the operative field. Ergonomically appropriate posture can be readily maintained at the surgical console. Appropriate settings can be preprogrammed into the console and permanently save such that the Robot can readily "recall" the size and habitus of a particular operating surgeon. Furthermore, the ability to perform tissue transfer in anatomical regions that are difficult to access will be greatly enhanced. Microsurgical intraoral reconstruction for malignant head and neck lesions has been performed with excellent success using a robotic telemanipulator [10]. Future organ transplantation may be enhanced by the ability to endoscopically access body cavities in minimally invasive fashion (Fig. 9.1).

The feasibility of performing microvascular anastomosis in an experimental model was demonstrated by Taleb et al. in 2008 [11]. They performed successful anastomosis of the tail artery of a rat utilizing the da Vinci Surgical Robot and 10-0 nylon suture. The authors concluded that the neutralization of physiological tremor, the simultaneous use of three instruments, the improved operator's gesture, and a very short learning curve made the application of this technique in human clinical practice a valuable prospect. Further experimentation was recommended.

Currently, the robotic surgical telemanipulators do not have the capability to perform osteotomy, osteoclasis, or osteosynthesis. However, combined traditional and robotic composite tissue transplant has been successful in an experimental model. This will be discussed in depth in a later chapter [12].

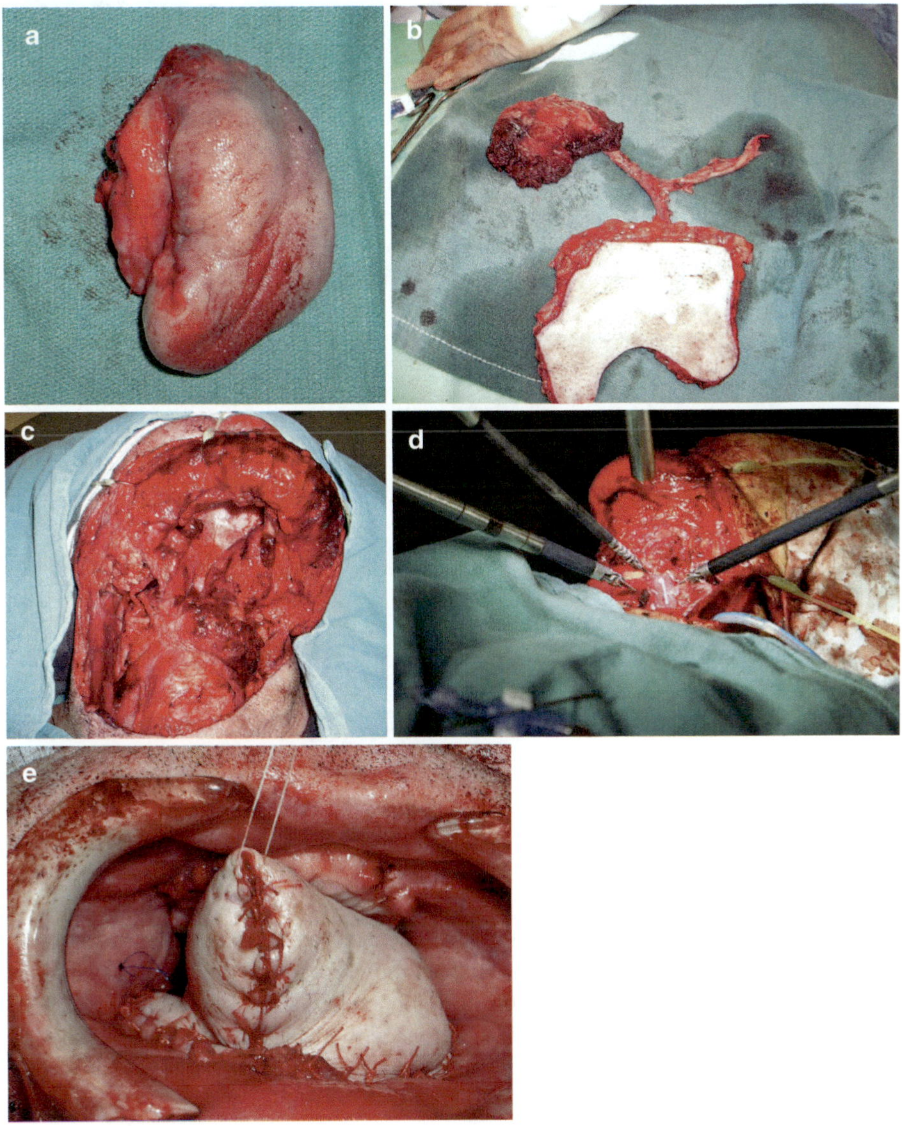

Fig. 9.1 Head and neck reconstruction. (**a**) Malignant lesion of tongue (**b**) Anterolateral thigh flap. (**c**) Intraoral recipient bed. (**d**) Robotic anastomosis of flap. (**e**) Tongue reconstruction completed

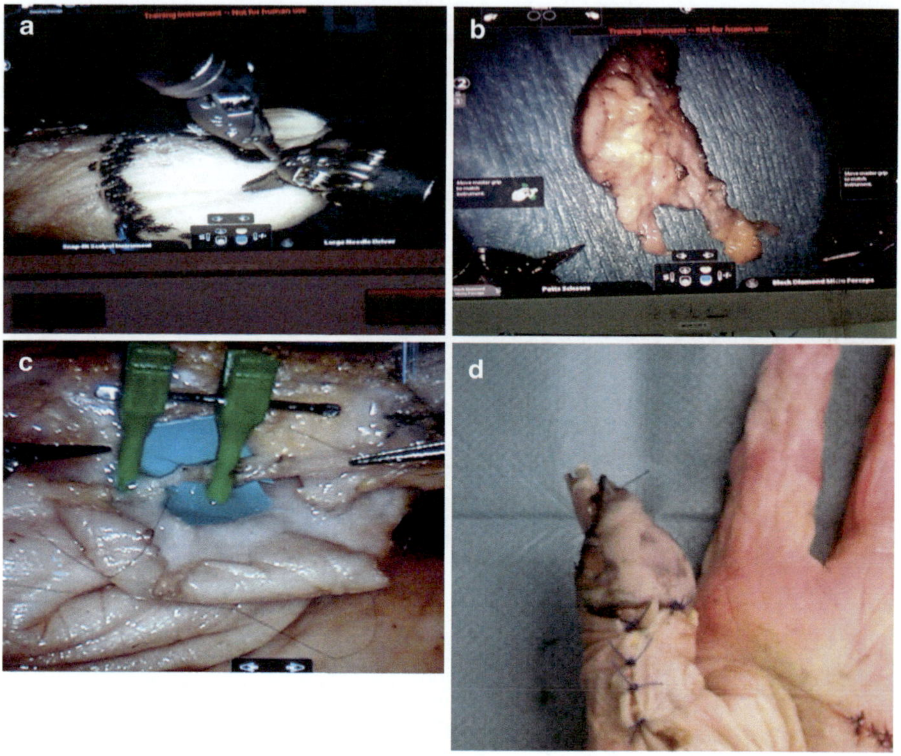

Fig. 9.2 Hand surgery. (**a**) Robotic harvest of great toe pulp. (**b**) Pulp of great toe with pedicle and attached skin as seen through robot console. (**c**) Anastomosis to thumb pedicle. (**d**) Insetting of flap completed

The feasibility of transferring of soft elements has been demonstrated in a laboratory model as well as clinically. An experimental free tissue transfer of skin, soft tissue, and vascular pedicle from the pulp of the great toe to the recipient denuded surface of the volar pad of the thumb was demonstrated at the second annual RASH (robotic-assisted surgery of the hand) society meeting IRCAD facility in Strasbourg, France, on March 4, 2010. This procedure was performed in its entirety using the da Vinci Robot (Fig. 9.2).

Conclusion

The cumulative preliminary results of the laboratory free tissue transfer experiments suggest that with high likelihood, transition to the clinical setting would be feasible. Early results in reconstructive head and neck cancer surgery are promising. Telemanipulator/robotic-assisted free tissue transfer holds great promise for the future, as the field of reconstructive microsurgery is poised to enter a new period of significant growth, as was noted in the 1960s and 1970s. The ultraprecise nature of microscopic robotic surgery will likely permit free tissue transfer on smaller, more delicate vascular pedicles and in locations that heretofore were inaccessible.

References

1. American Replantation Mission to China (1973) Replantation surgery in China. Plast Reconstr Surg 52:476–489
2. Chen C-W, Chien Y-C, Pao Y-S (1963) Salvage of the forearm following complete traumatic amputation: report of a case. Chin Med J 82:632
3. Cobbett JR (1969) Free digital transfer: report of a case of transfer of a great toe to replace an amputated thumb. J Bone Joint Surg Br 51B:677–679
4. Cohn LH (2006) Future directions in cardiac surgery. Am Heart Hosp J 4:174–178
5. Daniel RK, May JW Jr (1978) Free flaps: an overview. Clin Orthop 133:122–131
6. Jacobson JH, Suarez EI (1960) Microsurgery in anastomosis of small vessels. Surg Forum 11:243–245
7. Kleinert H, Kasdan M, Romero JL (1963) Small blood vessel anastomosis for salvage of severely injured upper extremity. J Bone Joint Surg Br 45A:788–796
8. Morrison WA, O'Brien BMC, MacLeod A (1978) Clinical experiences in free flap transfer. Clin Orthop 133:129–139
9. Nakayama K, Yamamoto K, Tamiya T et al (1964) Experience with free autografts of the bowel with a new venous anastomosis apparatus. Surgery 55:796–802
10. Selber J (2010) Transoral robotic reconstruction of oropharyngeal defects: a case series. Plast Reconstr Surg 126:1978–1987
11. Taleb C, Nectoux E, Liverneaux P (2009) Limb replantation with two robots: a feasibility study in a pig model. Microsurgery 29:232–235
12. Taleb C, Nectoux E, Liverneaux PA (2008) Telemicrosurgery: a feasibility study in a rat model. Chir Main 27:104–108

Tele-endomicrosurgery

10

Sybille Facca, Kiyohito Naito, Thierry Lequint, Eric Nectoux, and Philippe Liverneaux

10.1 Introduction

Characteristics of robots are well adapted to open telemicrosurgery: suppression of physiological tremor, optical magnification of the surgeon's movements, and improved ergonomics of the console. Previous chapters have well demonstrated that open telemicrosurgery is easily applicable to numerous surgical disciplines. Why not extend this concept to minimally invasive surgery, in order to operate in subcutaneous spaces by means of infracentimetric approaches? Similarly to laparoscopic telesurgery, trying to develop the surgical concept of tele-endomicrosurgery seems perfectly logical. Chapters 13 and 17 showed it was technically

S. Facca, M.D.
Department of Hand Surgery, Strasbourg University Hospitals, Illkirch, Strasbourg F-67403, France

K. Naito, M.D.
Department of Hand Surgery, Strasbourg University Hospitals, Illkirch, Strasbourg, F-67403, France

Department of Orthopaedics, Juntendo University, Tokyo, Japan

T. Lequint, M.D.
Department of Hand Surgery, Strasbourg University Hospitals, Illkirch, Strasbourg, F-67403, France

Department of Orthopaedics, Grand Hôpital, Charleroi, Belgium

E. Nectoux, M.D.
Department of Children's Surgery and Orthopaedics, Lille University Hospital, Lille 2 Nord de France University, Lille, France

P. Liverneaux, M.D., Ph.D. (✉)
Department of Hand Surgery, Strasbourg University Hospitals, Illkirch, Strasbourg F-67403, France

European Institute of TeleSurgery, IRCAD, Strasbourg, France
e-mail: philippe.liverneaux@chru-strasbourg.fr

P. Liverneaux et al. (eds.), *Telemicrosurgery*,
DOI 10.1007/978-2-8178-0391-3_10, © Springer-Verlag France 2013

possible to perform tele-endomicrosurgery of the brachial plexus by insufflation with carbon dioxide. The latter insufflation technique does not seem adapted to limb surgery as superficial aponeurosis on the one hand, and deep muscular compartments on the other hand do not allow sufficient visibility of vascular and nervous elements.

The aim of this chapter is to study the feasibility of limb tele-endomicrosurgery by means of a tele-endomicrosurgical median nerve repair model in the forearm, using a specific surgical retractor.

10.2 Material and Methods

The material consisted of a fresh defrosted human cadaver forearm, a da Vinci SI® robot (Intuitive Surgical™, Sunnyvale, CA, USA), a retractor specifically designed for tele-endomicrosurgery by IiN Medical™ (Besançon, France) (Fig. 10.1).

The forearm was placed in the supine position, the body of the robot on the radial aspect of the limb, and the instruments being the ulnar side.

Five approaches were prepared, one small puncture for the insertion of the retractor, a one-centimeter incision for the camera, and three separate 8-mm-long incisions for instrumentation (Fig. 10.2a). All approaches converged toward a central cavity (or working chamber) created with dissecting scissors anterior to the median nerve. The specialized retractor was spread to maintain sufficient space inside the working chamber (Fig. 10.2b). The four trocars were fixed to the arms of the robot (Fig. 10.2c).

The median nerve was dissected and pulled from the underlying tissues by a surgical loop (Fig. 10.3a), then an experimental laceration of the median nerve was performed in the distal third of the forearm (Fig. 10.3b). Suture repair was performed with epiperineural stitches of 10/0 nylon using two Black Diamond® forceps and Potts® scissors (Intuitive Surgical™, Sunnyvale, CA, USA) (Fig. 10.3c). Suture quality was assessed by mobilizing the repaired nervous segment with a Maryland® forceps (Intuitive Surgical™, Sunnyvale, CA, USA).

10.3 Results

Tele-endomicrosurgical suture of the median nerve presented no particular technical problem (video). However, several difficulties were encountered while performing the approach to the median nerve.

The first difficulty concerned the working chamber. Its realization included two steps, one superficial and one deep. The superficial step did not prove difficult, whether for the creation of the chamber or its maintenance with the specific retractor. The deep dissection into the anterior muscular compartment of the forearm was much more difficult, first because it was challenging to locate the median nerve without any visible anatomical landmarks, and second because it was challenging to

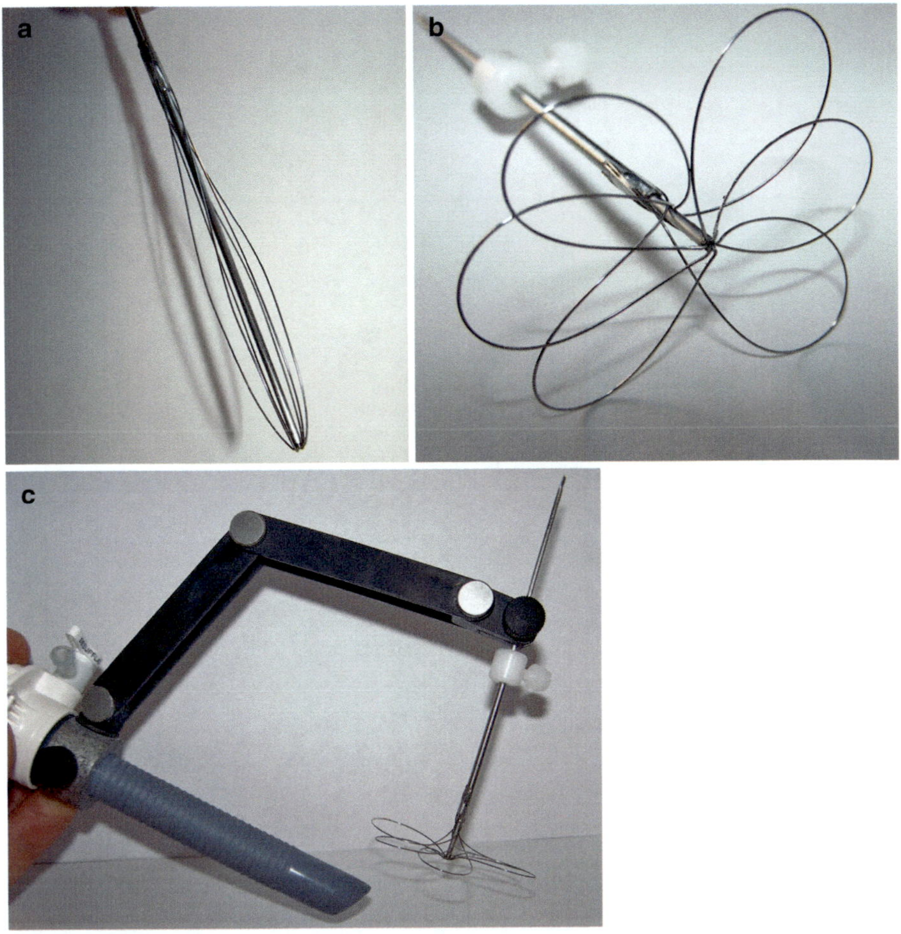

Fig. 10.1 Specific retractor designed to maintain a working chamber during a tele-endomicrosurgical median nerve repair at the forearm: (**a**) Closed specific retractor. (**b**) Spread specific retractor. (**c**) Specific retractor fixed to the optical trocar of the da Vinci® robot by an articulated arm

maintain a sufficiently wide perineural working chamber. The specific retractor could not maintain a working chamber around the nerve. A Maryland® forceps was used for this purpose.

The second difficulty was represented by both instrumental and optical trocars. In laparoscopic telesurgery, da Vinci® trocars should be inserted a minimum of 8 cm inside the abdomen to prevent accidental extraction which would render the surgical procedure impossible. In the forearm, this 8 cm distance is quite large regarding the relatively small size of the compartment and close relationships among the anatomical structures. Therefore, it was compulsory to frequently assess the position of the trocars throughout the entire surgical procedure.

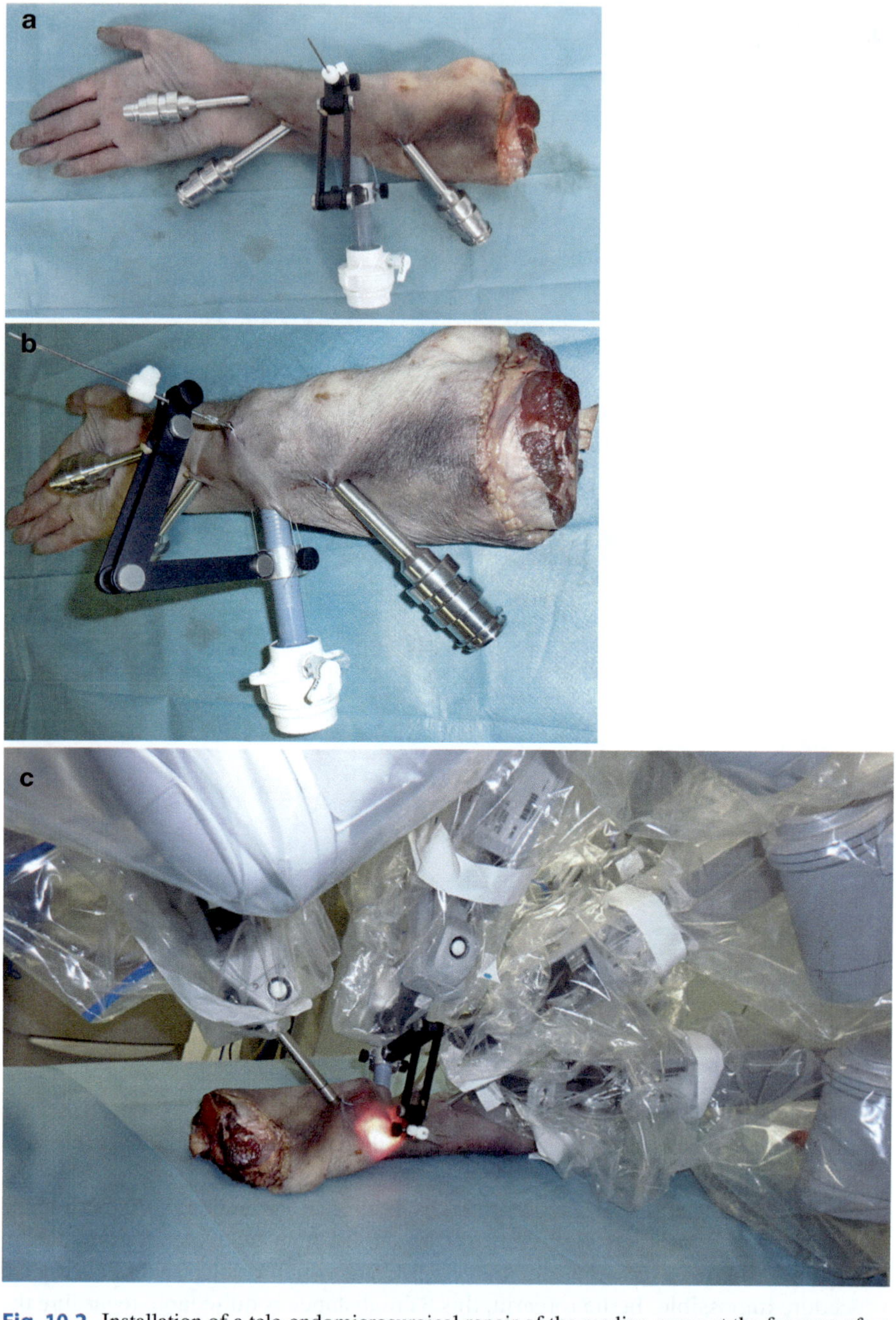

Fig. 10.2 Installation of a tele-endomicrosurgical repair of the median nerve at the forearm of an anatomical subject. (**a**) Trocars converge toward the working chamber. The central trocar is for the 3D camera. Lateral trocars allow the instruments of the robot. (**b**) The specific retractor fixed to the optical trocar is spread inside the working chamber. (**c**) The trocars are adapted to the robot's arms onto which are fixed the 3D camera and three instruments

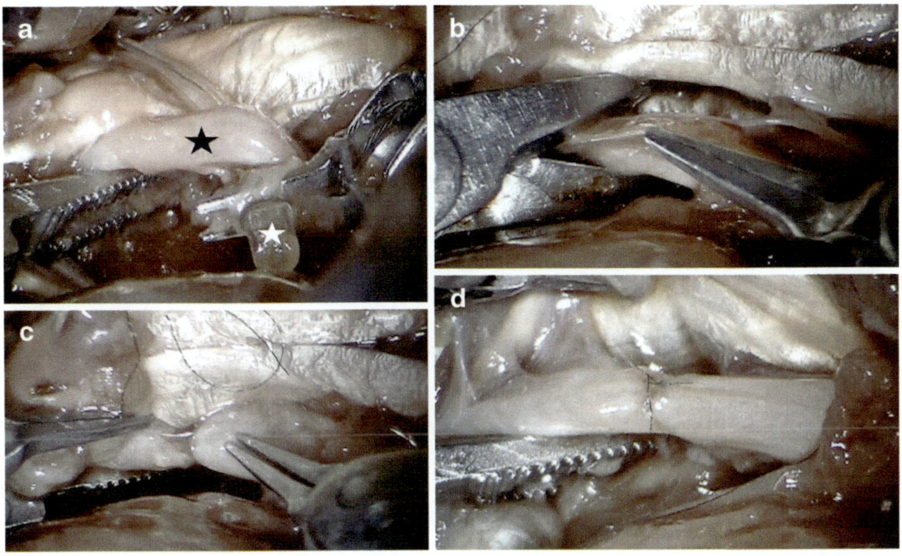

Fig. 10.3 Master-console screen view of a tele-endomicrosurgical repair of the median nerve at the forearm in an anatomical subject: (**a**) Median nerve (*black star*) is marked by a surgical loop (*white star*). (**b**) Section of the median nerve using Potts® scissors. (**c**) Epiperineural stitching of the nervous section with 10/0 nylon. (**d**) Final aspect of the nervous repair

The third difficulty came from the blurriness of the camera vision, due to the quickly rising temperature inside the working chamber. This problem was solved by adding a small suction device through another instrumental trocar.

Navigating the instruments across the metallic threads of the specialized retractor proved challenging, and this fourth difficulty was solved by manipulating the metallic threads of the retractor with the robot's instruments.

Finally, the fifth difficulty followed from the fourth, as a supplemental instrument was required to spread either the metallic threads of the retractor or the surrounding muscles and could therefore not be used to help with the microsurgical repair.

10.4 Discussion

Peripheral nerve, vascular and tendinous surgery could very well benefit from and evolve toward less invasive techniques.

On reading our results, it seems that a tele-endomicrosurgery feasibility concept has been demonstrated. However, an attempt at experimental analysis of such a concept highlights the need for specific instrumentation not only to create and maintain a proper working chamber but also to manipulate anatomical structures with ever more precise instruments. The robot itself should evolve and the configuration of a da Vinci® robot is not adapted yet to tele-endomicrosurgery. The "single port" concept in laparoscopic surgery is starting to grow and could very well become a gold standard in the future [1].

Reference

1. Kaouk JH, Goel RK, Haber GP (2009) Robotic single-port trans-umbilical surgery in humans: initial report. BJU Int 103:366–369

Brachial Plexus Repair

11

Gustavo Mantovani Ruggiero and Philippe Liverneaux

11.1 Introduction

Modern concept of peripheral nerve repair was described in the late nineteenth century. Survival rates after severe upper and lower extremity injuries improved during the Second World War. Seddon's observations and research served as a guide for treating nerve injuries [12, 15, 16]. In the latter part of the twentieth century, Millesi recognized the necessity of matching thc internal fascicles of nerves [8, 9, 10]. Sunderland described the concept of interfascicular nerve grafting [16–18]. Gentle handling of the stumps of injured nerves and meticulous suturing of the various layers that compose the peripheral nerve is well described and is associated with reliable clinical results. The repair can be performed as an end-to-end suture, between the nerve epineurium, perineurium, or a combination of both layers. Nerve gaps can be reconstructed through nerve grafts or neurotubes [1].

Technical limitations effect the results of nerve repair. Impediments to restoration of neural function can relate to imprecision of the anastomosis. Inadequate matching of motor and sensory fibers in mixed nerves can produce nonfunctioning cross-connections, thus limiting transmission of appropriate neural signals to the target organs. Precise suture connection using Millesi's perineural suture technique of matching fascicles according to size and location within the nerve may increase clinical success [11].

G.M. Ruggiero, M.D. (✉)
Department of Hand Surgery, São Paulo Hand Center,
Beneficiencia Portuguesa de Sao Paulo Hospital,
Rua Maestro Cardim, 987, Sao Paolo 01323-001, Brazil
e-mail: mantovani@sphandcenter.com

P. Liverneaux, M.D., Ph.D.
Department of Hand Surgery, Strasbourg University Hospitals,
F-67403 Illkirch, France

European Institute of TeleSurgery, IRCAD,
F-67000 Strasbourg, France

P. Liverneaux et al. (eds.), *Telemicrosurgery*,
DOI 10.1007/978-2-8178-0391-3_11, © Springer-Verlag France 2013

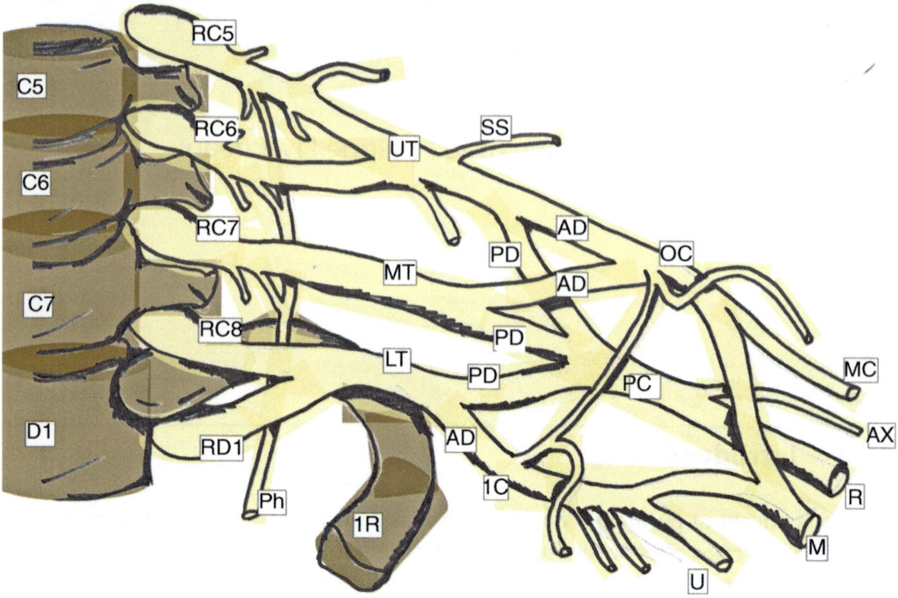

Fig. 11.1 Schematic anatomy of brachial plexus. Bone structures (*C5-C6-C7-D1* 5th to 7th cervical spine vertebraes and 1st dorsal spine vertebrae, *1R* 1st rib). Brachial plexus components (*RC5-RC8* 5th to 8th cervical brachial plexus roots, *RD1* 1st dorsal brachial plexus root, *UT* upper trunk, *MT* middle trunk, *LT* lower trunk, *PD* posterior division from each trunk, *AD* anterior division from each trunk, *OC* outer chord, *PC* posterior chord, *IC* inner chord). Main nerve branches (*Ph* phrenic nerve, *SS* suprascapular nerve, *MC* musculocutaneous nerve, *Ax* axillary nerve, *R* radial nerve, *M* median nerve, *U* ulnar nerve)

These principles can be applied, in general, to any peripheral nerve repair. However, there are specific anatomic sites where greater complexity of the neural elements are encountered. These sites are the plexiform formation of the emerging nerves on the cervical spine (brachial plexus) or lumbosacral spine (lumbar-sacral plexus).

The brachial plexus is an intricate web-like nervous formation that emerges from the C4 to T1 vertebral levels. Several interneural crossing connections occur within the cervical, supra, and infraclavicular regions. The brachial plexus is the origin of all nervous branches that provide the sensory and motor innervation of the upper limb (Fig. 11.1) [8].

The most frequent injuries affecting the brachial plexus are closed traumatic traction lesions, often related to high-energy accidents affecting young adults. In addition, newborn upper limb palsy may also occur as a result of brachial plexus during a traumatic delivery [3, 21].

Open injuries by gunshots or penetrating trauma are less common. These injuries are often associated with serious vascular injuries which frequently require urgent restoration of circulation. This subset of combined vascular and neurologic brachial plexus injuries is subject to a multidisciplinary approach and therefore is excluded from this discussion.

The complex anatomy of the brachial plexus represents a series of challenges for the surgeon. In addition to identifying the origin and pathway of the injured neural structures, it is important to reestablish orientation of the damaged branches to enhance precise matching of motor and sensory branches [3].

In those injuries affecting branch points of the brachial plexus, it can be difficult or impossible to accurately reestablish the proper anatomic pathways. In such circumstances, the use of nerve grafts or neurotubes may be beneficial. The connections are promoted by chemotaxis which may enhance union of the nerve endings, but cross-linking can occur resulting in a diminished recovery of function [3].

Some unreconstructible injuries may require a different strategy. Options include the various neurotization techniques. This consists of the transfer of functional nerves to the injured distal stumps of the brachial plexus components [4, 13]. Common donor site nerves are the accessory nerve (XI cranial nerve), the intercostal nerves, or motor fascicles of a noninjured nerve as in the Oberlin technique [4, 13].

11.2 Robot-Assisted Brachial Plexus Surgery

Traditionally, the diagnosis and treatment of closed brachial plexus injuries is dictated, primarily, by clinical examination. A meticulous physical exam can be used to define the components of the plexus affected by the trauma; however, it is not possible to differentiate between neurotmesis, axonotmesis, or neuropraxia. Unfortunately, these degrees of injury cannot be differentiated accurately by any imaging examination, nor by electromyography (EMG). As such, severity of injury can be gauged through serial clinical examinations during the first 2–3 months after the trauma. Clinical evolution, or lack thereof, helps further define the lesion [2, 3].

Serial examination is useful in determining candidacy for surgical intervention. However, this approach can be accompanied by a delay in exploration of 3–6 months post-injury. This adds a critical degree of difficulty to the surgery, as exposure and exploration of the plexus and its components requires dissection through scar tissue around and within the neural structures.

11.2.1 Quality Improvement of the Nerve Repair

Robot-assisted surgery for brachial plexus trauma may improve the quality of the nerve repair. The features of the robot-assisted microsurgery that create an ideal environment for a successful repair are high definition 3D vision, excellent ergonomics for the surgeon, amplification of the range of motion of the instruments, and amplification of the precision of those movements.

Various experimental models were used in the initial robotic microsurgical trials to simulate clinical situations. These included earthworm anastomoses, chicken thigh arterial and venous repair, rat sciatic nerve repair, and complex procedures such as complete limbs replantations in pigs [6, 11, 19, 20]. Microsurgical procedures require manipulation of ultrafine suture material, such as 8-0, 9-0, and 10-0 nylon. An initial barrier to acceptance of the robot as a useful device for assisting in microsurgery was the concern held by some surgeons regarding the lack of haptic feedback from the telemanipulator systems available. The initial experimental experience suggested that there was no difficulty manipulating fine suture material with the robot, suggesting that haptic sensation was not necessary. This was further confirmed by an interesting and simple study showing that most experienced microsurgeons are not able to feel the haptic feedback when performing conventional microsurgery [14].

Clinical use of the robotic telemanipulation was introduced to perform nerve repair by Philippe Liverneaux in France in 2009, by Stacey Berner in the USA in 2010, and by Gustavo Mantovani Ruggiero in Brazil in 2011. Initially, the robot was used in place of the conventional microscope, after a traditional open dissection technique. When the surgery reached the point where the nerve suture repair or reconstruction was required, instead of installing the microscope, the robot was docked into the operating field and the surgeon performed the nerve suture from the surgeon's console of the equipment. This technique was successfully utilized to perform brachial plexus repair (Fig. 11.2) and to treat other peripheral nerve injuries on the upper and lower limbs. The ability to perform successful repair was confirmed, but the entire potential of robot-assisted microneural surgery was not realized during these initial cases. The instrumentation used on the earliest experimental and clinical cases was not specifically designed to microsurgery. Similarly, the magnification and optical capabilities were not designed for this purpose. The equipment available, the da Vinci® system (Intuitive Surgical™, Sunnyvale, CA, USA), was mainly designed for laparoscopic surgery. Therefore, there is vast potential for the future development of refined technology, providing more appropriate forceps, graspers, welding techniques, fibrin glue injection techniques, and improvement in the magnification. Ultimately, this may create the conditions to perform "nerve super-microsurgery." The ability to utilize ultrahigh magnification to manipulate individual fascicles inside the nerves would result in highly precise connections [5].

11.2.2 Mini-Invasive Approach

The feasibility of performing nerve repair with robotic telemanipulation has been confirmed. A secondary application and potential benefit of robotic manipulation is the ability to perform for nerve surgery using a minimally invasive approach.

A challenge in performing minimally invasive procedures is providing necessary space to see and manipulate the structures. This is easily obtained in the natural anatomic cavities of human body, such as the abdominal and thoracic cavity, but is a barrier when dealing with the extremities (upper and lower limbs).

The brachial plexus has some unique anatomical relationships which render minimally invasive procedures possible. The supraclavicular fossa acts as a cavity, and gas insufflation with low pressure is adequate to elevate the subcutaneous and skin away from deeper structures. Similar structural relationships have not yet been completely defined elsewhere in the extremities, although research is ongoing.

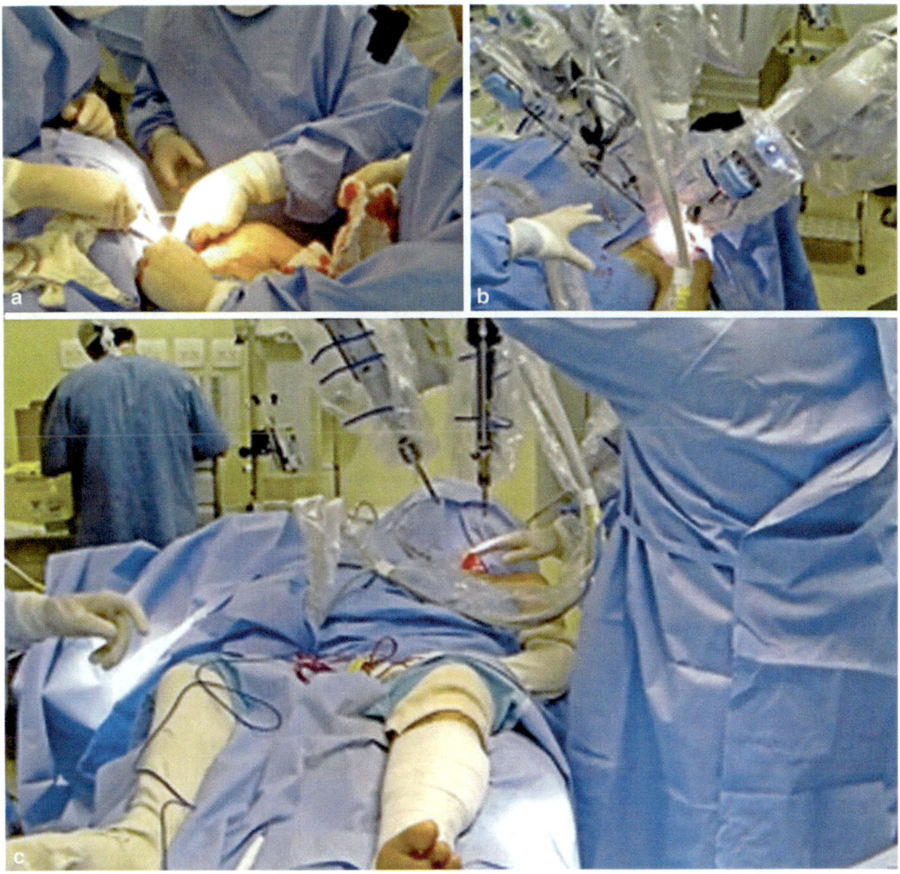

Fig. 11.2 Clinical use of the robot on a brachial plexus injury repair using a traditional open approach. (**a**) Dissection of the brachial plexus by traditional open approach. (**b**, **c**) Docking of the robot behind the patient and positioning of the robot camera and arms on the operating field

Based on the potential capacity to create a cavity adjacent to the brachial plexus and the feasibility of manipulation of this nervous structure with the robot, an experimental study was designed with the objective of creating a robot-assisted minimally invasive endoscopic approach to the human brachial plexus [7].

The experimental model used a fresh human cadaver for this research. The technique employed three portals along the clavicular line, a central portal for the robot 3D camera and the two side portals for the robot telemanipulated arms (Fig. 11.3). A complete dissection and full exposure of the supraclavicular portion of the brachial plexus was successfully achieved in this experiment (Fig. 11.4). Reconstruction of an experimentally created upper trunk lesion was performed with similar facility to the previously noted clinical cases. The improvement of natural range of motion and precision of the surgeon's movements allowed the investigator to perform an epineural suture with nerve graft in the small cavity space created by the gas

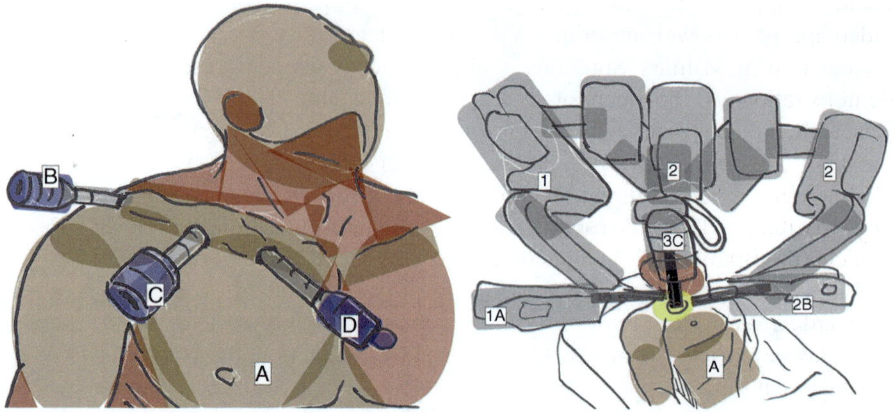

Fig. 11.3 Schematic illustration of the endoscopic exploration of brachial plexus using the da Vinci Robot. *A* – Human fresh cadaver. *B* – First cannula and portal to robot arm. *C* – Cannula and portal for robot camera. *D* – Second cannula and portal to robot arm; *1, 2, 3* robot components to move the instrument's arms and camera, *1A* and *2B* robot instruments, *3C* robot 3D camera and optics

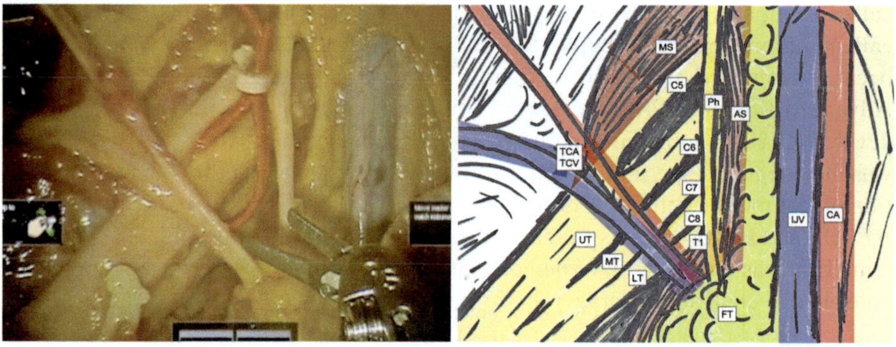

Fig. 11.4 Endoscopic view of brachial plexus through the robot camera (*TCA* transverse cervical artery, *TCV* transverse cervical vein, *MS* medium scalene muscle, *AS* anterior scalene muscle, *IJV* internal jugular vein, *CA* carotid artery, *FT* fat tissue, *Ph* phrenic nerve, *C5-T1* brachial plexus roots, *UT* upper trunk, *MT* middle trunk, *LT* lower trunk)

insufflation (Fig. 11.5). This first experiment was recently published on the scientific literature [7] and opened the pathway to the first clinical trials and potentially may alter the approach to management of closed brachial plexus injuries.

11.2.3 Early Diagnosis of Brachial Plexus Injuries Lesions

A concern regarding the clinical application of minimally invasive reconstructive procedures for brachial plexus injury is the dissection through the scar tissue. It can be tedious and difficult to dissect and identify the neural components within the

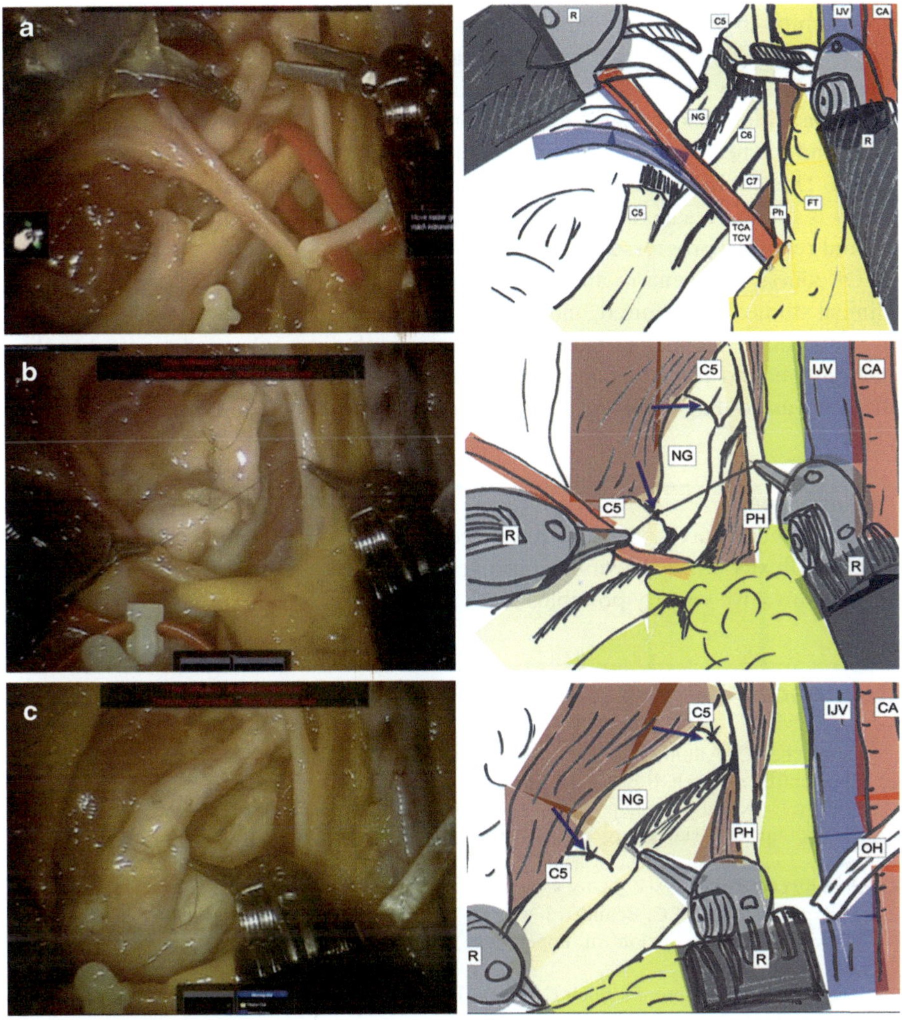

Fig. 11.5 Endoscopic view of brachial plexus through the robot camera proceeding a nerve graft to C5 reconstruction. (**a**) C5 gap with the nerve graft positioned. (**b**) Robot instruments performing the epineural suture. (**c**) Nerve grafting for C5 reconstruction done (*R* robot instruments, *IJV* internal jugular vein, *CA* carotid artery, *FT* fat tissue, *TCA, TCV* transverse cervical artery and vein, *C5* C5 root, *NG* nerve graft, *Ph* phrenic nerve, *OH* omohyoid tendon cut; *blue arrows*: suture knots with 9-0 nylon to epineural suture)

fibrous scar tissue when doing a traditional open approach. However, the robot assisted endoscopic approach may provide an alternative to the traditional "watch and wait" approach. As noted in the previous discussion, historically, delayed exploration has been employed by many surgeons. We believe the endoscopic robot-assisted approach may be used in the future for diagnosis and treatment for acute injuries of the brachial plexus. Those who treat these complex injuries may have the opportunity, to perform a minimally invasive procedure, of no more than 30 min of surgical time, with minimal blood loss and limited inducement of scar formation. This could allow exploration and visualization of the entire supraclavicular portion of the brachial plexus. Early exploration of closed brachial plexus injuries in the adult and the newborn with an Erb-Duchenne Palsy could confirm the nature of the lesion. This could permit immediate treatment, or in the case where no macroscopic injury is found, less anxiety and doubt to patients, therapists, doctors, and family as natural recovery progresses.

Of course the scenario above is not a prompt reality. Further experimental and clinical studies are required, and some drawbacks are expected. However, advances of the robotic telemanipulation technology including enhanced tissue handling instruments and retractors may improve the facility of performing prompt minimally invasive diagnosis and treatment of brachial plexus injuries in the years to come.

Conclusion

In the near future, robot-assisted surgery may provide an early diagnosis of brachial plexus injuries lesions, improve the quality of the nerve repair, and make mini-invasive surgery possible.

References

1. Desouches C, Alluin O, Mutaftschiev N et al (2005) Peripheral nerve repair: 30 centuries of scientific research. Rev Neurol (Paris) 161:1045–1059
2. Giuffre JL, Kakar S, Bishop AT et al (2010) Current concepts of the treatment of adult brachial plexus injuries. J Hand Surg 35A:678–688
3. Isaacs J (2010) Treatment of acute peripheral nerve injuries: current concepts. J Hand Surg 35A:491–497
4. Liverneaux P, Diaz LC, Beaulieu J-Y et al (2006) Preliminary results of double nerve transfer to restore elbow flexion in upper type brachial plexus palsies. Plast Reconstr Surg 117:915–919
5. Liverneaux P, Nectoux E, Taleb C (2009) The future of robotics in hand surgery. Chir Main 28:278–285
6. Mantovani G, Fukushima WY, Baik Cho A, Aita MA, Mazzetti MV (2009) Use of earthworms for microsurgery training. J Reconstr Microsurg 25:275–278
7. Mantovani G, Liverneaux P, Garcia JC et al (2011) Endoscopic exploration and repair of brachial plexus with telerobotic manipulation: a cadaver trial. J Neurosurg 8:1–6
8. Millesi H (1984) The current state of peripheral nerve surgery in the upper limb. Ann Chir Main 3:18–34
9. Millesi H (1986) The nerve gap. Theory and clinical practice. Hand Clin 2:651–663
10. Millesi H (2006) Factors affecting the outcome of peripheral nerve surgery. Microsurgery 26:295–302
11. Nectoux E, Taleb C, Liverneaux P (2009) Nerve repair in telemicrosurgery: an experimental study. J Reconstr Microsurg 25:261–265
12. Nicholson OR, Seddon HJ (1957) Nerve repair in civil practice; results of treatment of median and ulnar nerve lesions. Br Med J 9:1065–1071
13. Oberlin C, Durand S, Belheyar Z et al (2009) Nerve transfers in brachial plexus palsies. Chir Main 28:1–9

14. Panchulidze I, Berner S, Mantovani G et al (2011) Is haptic feedback necessary to microsurgical suturing? Comparative study of 9/0 and 10/0 knot tying operated by 24 surgeons. Hand Surg 16:1–3
15. Seddon H (1968) Advances in nerve repair. Triangle 8:252–259
16. Sunderland S (1953) Funicular suture and funicular exclusion in the repair of severed nerves. Br J Surg 40:580–587
17. Sunderland S (1979) Advances in diagnosis and treatment of root and peripheral nerve injury. Adv Neurol 22:271–305
18. Sunderland S (1981) The anatomic foundation of peripheral nerve repair techniques. Orthop Clin North Am 12:245–266
19. Taleb C, Nectoux E, Liverneaux PA (2008) Telemicrosurgery: a feasibility study in a rat model. Chir Main 27:104–108
20. Taleb C, Nectoux E, Liverneaux P (2009) Limb replantation with two robots: a feasibility study in a pig model. Microsurgery 29:232–235
21. Zafeiriou DI, Psychogiou K (2008) Obstetrical brachial plexus palsy. Pediatr Neurol 38:235–242

12 Tendon Transfer

Michael S. Bednar

12.1 Introduction

> In muscle tendon surgery there is very little hope that errors in technique can be overcome by local adaptation. The success or failure of an operation depends upon the technical competence of the operator and his painstaking after-care. —Paul Riordan

One of the main advantages of using the surgical robot for is minimizing surgical scar. In tendon transfer procedures, one of the tenets of successful surgery is to place the transferred tendon in an unscarred bed to prevent adhesions. Yet in many tendon transfer procedures, large incisions are placed directly over the site of the tendon transfer. This chapter reviews basic principles of tendon transfer procedures and then demonstrates the advantage of dissection of the donor muscle with the surgical robot in tendon transfer procedures.

In a tendon transfer procedure, the terminal end of a tendon connected to a voluntarily activated muscle is transected at its insertion and then woven into the tendon of a nonfunctional tendon-muscle unit. Loss of function may be from an injury to the brain (cerebral palsy, stroke), to the upper motor neurons (spinal cord injury), to the lower motor neurons (peripheral nerve palsy, leprosy, Charcot-Marie-Tooth), to the muscles (arthrogryposis), to the tendon (chronic tendon laceration/avulsion), or from a combination (trauma). The goal of the procedure is to produce voluntary, active motion in the paralyzed region of the limb.

M.S. Bednar, M.D.
Orthopaedic Surgery and Rehabilitation, Stritch School of Medicine,
Loyola University, 1700 Maguire Building, 2160 S. First Avenue,
Maywood 60153, IL, USA
e-mail: mbednar@lumc.edu

P. Liverneaux et al. (eds.), *Telemicrosurgery*,
DOI 10.1007/978-2-8178-0391-3_12, © Springer-Verlag France 2013

12.2 Prerequisites

Patients considered for tendon transfer procedures must have expendable muscles that are available for transfer (donor muscle) [1]. Expendable means that there is more than one muscle that performs the same function (e.g., extensor carpi radialis longus ECRL and brevis ECRB are both radial wrist extensors). A donor muscle can be voluntarily controlled, is neither spastic nor injured, and must have adequate strength and excursion to perform the function of the paralyzed muscle. The strength of a muscle is proportional to the physiologic cross section of all muscle fibers, not the cross section of the muscle itself [8]. In this way, a multipennate muscle, with fibers directed in multiple orientations, is stronger than a unipennate muscle. Likewise, the excursion of a muscle is proportional of the length of the muscle fiber, not the length of the muscle itself.

Excursion of the muscle is the distance the terminal tendon end will travel from complete distraction (when the muscle is maximally pulled) to complete contraction. Digital flexors have an excursion of approximately 7 cm, digital extensors approximately 5 cm, and wrist motors approximately 3 cm. No tendon transfer can reproduce the excursion of the digital flexors, and transferring a wrist flexor cannot restore the complete excursion of the finger extensors. However, the excursion of any transfers can be improved by moving the intercalary joints. In the example of finger extension, the transfer must be set loosely enough that the fingers can be passively brought into full flexion with the wrist in extension. As such, there is not enough excursion of the transferred muscle to extend the fingers with the wrist in extension. However, flexing the wrist joint improves excursion of the transfer to the digital extensors via the tenodesis effect. For patients to gain maximum finger extension after a tendon transfer of a wrist flexor to the digital extensor tendons, the wrist needs to be in partial flexion.

The excursion of a transferred muscle can be increased in two additional ways. Transfers placed closer from the axis of rotation of the joint will have a larger excursion, but will have decreased force secondary to a larger lever arm. Excursion of some muscles can be improved by freeing their muscle fibers from connective tissue. Kozin and Bednar published on the excursion of the brachioradialis [7]. When the insertion of the muscle alone is transected and the muscle is maximally stimulated, the excursion was 8 mm. When the tendon was freed of soft tissue attachments to the musculotendinous junction, the excursion improved to 14 mm. When the muscle was freed of soft tissue attachments to the neurovascular insertion, the excursion improved to 61 mm. It has been hypothesized that the cost of increased excursion by this dissection may be loss of muscle force [9].

The other principles of tendon transfer are that the transfers should pass in a straight line. If the transfer needs to change direction, the pulley should be stable and straight. The concept of one muscle – one function means that you cannot expect one transfer to flex the interphalangeal joint of the thumb and extend the metacarpohalangeal joint of the index finger at the same time. When a transfer is

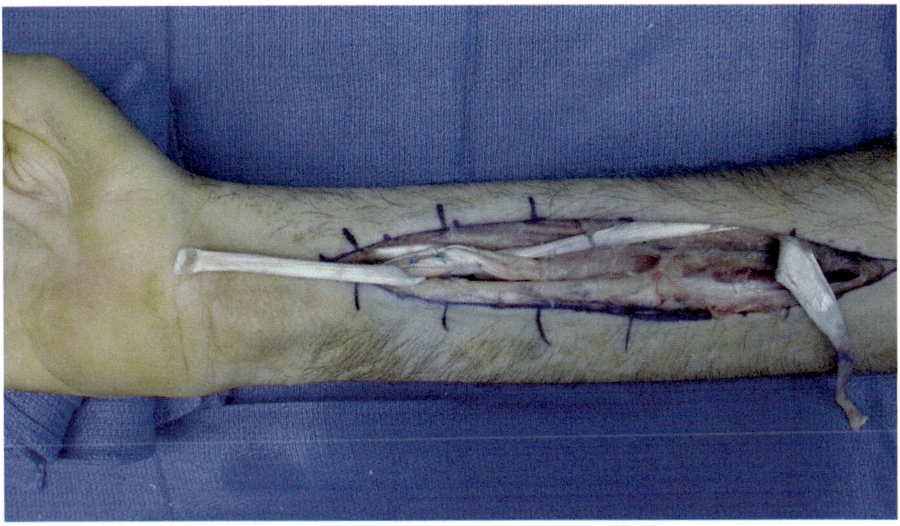

Fig. 12.1 Incision for tendon transfers for finger and thumb flexion. The transfer of the extensor carpi radialis to flexor digitorum profundus has been completed. The cut tendon of the brachioradialis is seen in preparation for transfer to the flexor pollicis longus. Note the long length of the incision and the immediate proximity of the tendon to the surgical incision

sewn into two insertions that perform different function, it will predominantly act on the tighter insertion. The limb should have bony stability (healed fractures) and mobile, stable joints. All edema and inflammation from trauma should be resolved. There must be an adequate soft tissue bed for the tendon transfer to glide in. Ideally, transfers should pass thru subcutaneous fat or between a fascial plane and subcutaneous fat. Tendon transfers cannot be placed under split thickness skin grafts.

Despite the knowledge that tendon transfers should ideally be placed in a scar free plane, many transfers are done immediately under the skin incision made to dissect the muscle from its facial attachments. When performing tendon transfers in the upper extremity in patients with tetraplegia, one of the most common procedures is to transfer the brachioradialis to the flexor pollicis longus to restore active pinch [2–6]. Exposure is through an incision along the radial or palmar-radial forearm, beginning at the wrist crease and extending between 10 and 20 cm proximally. The brachioradialis is detached from fascial attachment for a distance of 6–10 cm proximal to the musculotendinous junction. In the distal end of the incision, the deep flexor fascia is opened and the brachioradialis tendon is woven into flexor pollicis longus FPL tendon 2–3 cm distal to its musculotendinous junction. At the end of the procedure, the dissected brachioradialis muscle and tendon transfer site are immediately subcutaneous, directly under the surgical scar (Fig. 12.1). Adhesions between the skin and transferred tendon have been seen postoperatively. While the operation predictably restores pinch strength, the question remains as to whether the excursion

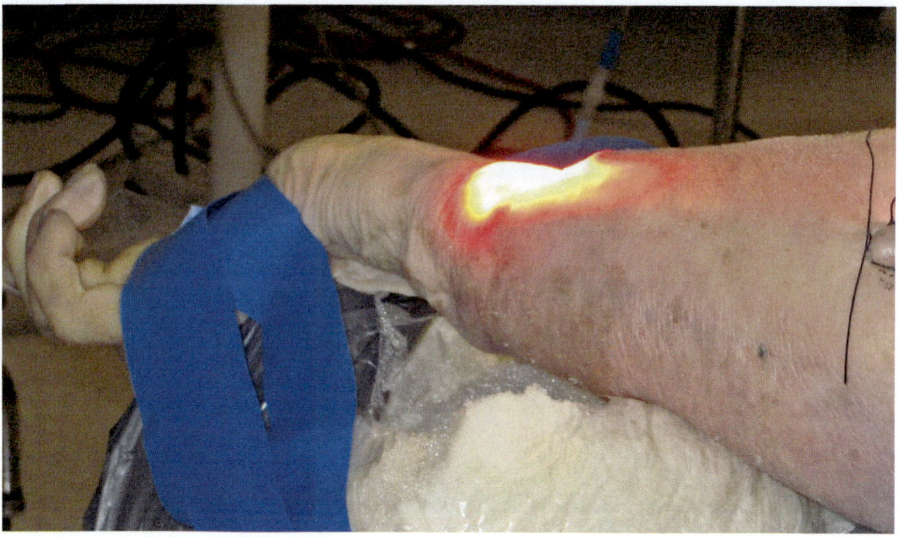

Fig. 12.2 Portals for tendon transfer in forearm, ulnar view

of the transfer and the pinch strength would be improved if the transfer could be done without a large skin incision in direct contact with the dissected muscle and tendons. In addition, patient acceptance of the procedure may be greater if it could be done through portal incisions rather than through a long vertical incision.

12.3 Robot-Assisted Tendon Transfer Procedure

There are no reports in the literature of using robotic surgery to perform tendon transfer procedures in the upper extremity. To test the feasibility of the procedure, two fresh cadavers were used. In each arm the da Vinci® Robot (Intuitive Surgical™, Sunnyvale, CA, USA) was used to circumferentially dissect the brachioradialis from its insertion at the distal radius to the junction of the proximal and middle thirds of the forearm. Three portals, each 1.5-cm long, were made for the camera, scissors, and forceps. Portals were placed 2–3 cm apart, beginning just distal to the medial epicondyle and moving radially (Figs. 12.2 and 12.3). Each instrument was placed through an insufflation cannula. Excellent visualization of the brachioradialis, ECRL and ECRB tendons, and the radial artery and superficial branch of the radial nerve was attained (Fig. 12.4). The fascia of the brachioradialis was dissected circumferential from the distal two-thirds of the muscle. The FPL tendon was then identified and longitudinally split distal to the musculotendinous junction (Fig. 12.5). The brachioradialis was detached from its insertion and was passed through the split

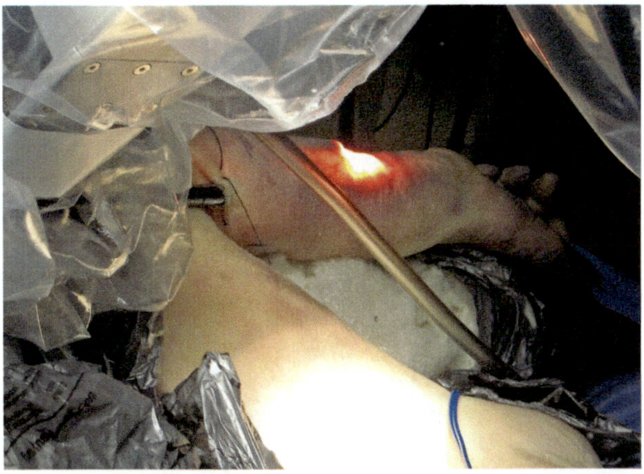

Fig. 12.3 Portals for tendon transfer in forearm, radial view

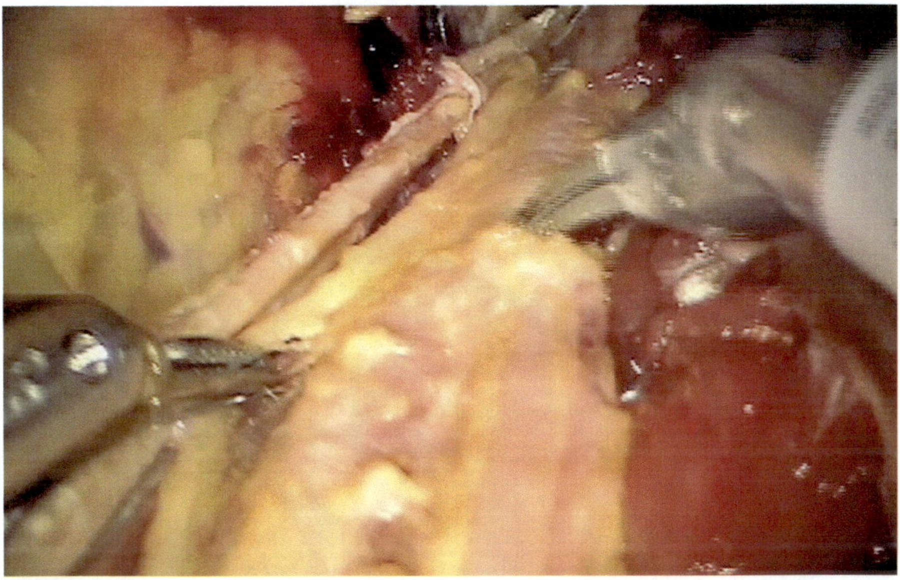

Fig. 12.4 View from the robotic camera. The four structures visualized from left to right are the tendon of the brachioradialis, the superficial branch of the radial nerve, the radial artery, and the tendon of the flexor pollicis longus

FPL tendon (Fig. 12.6). With the robot, sutures were placed through the distal end of the brachioradialis tendon. A fourth 1.5-cm incision was made at the site of the transfer to pass this suture outside of the skin. Tension was applied through the suture and the tendon transfer was sewn at the weave between the brachioradialis and flexor pollicis longus using the surgical robot.

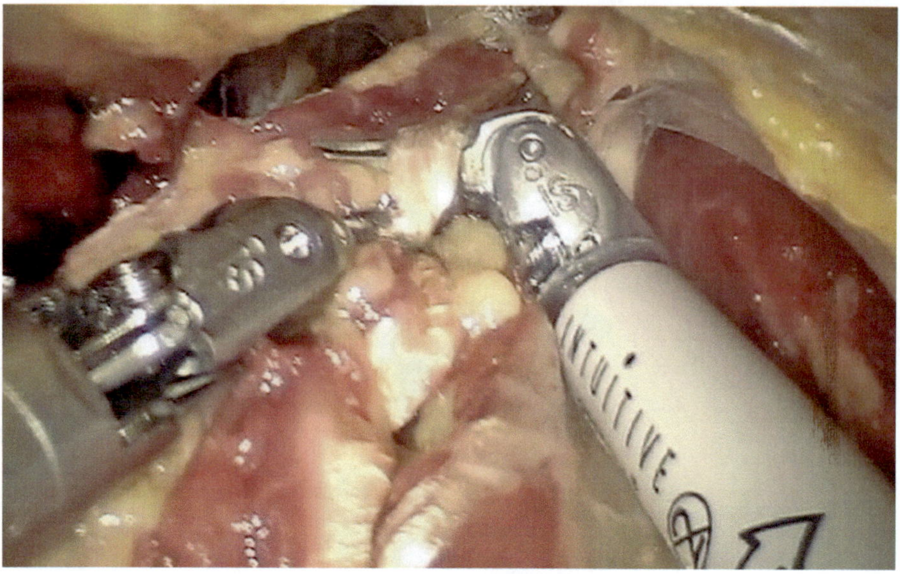

Fig. 12.5 Robotic scissors placed in the tendon of the flexor pollicis longus

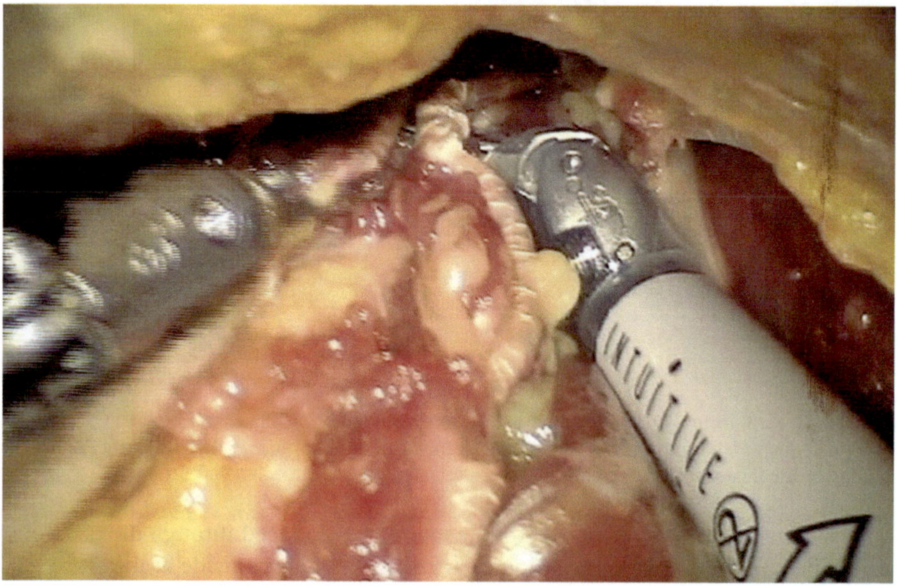

Fig. 12.6 Tendon of the brachioradialis brought against the flexor pollicis longus in preparation for tendon weave

Conclusions

The concept of harvesting muscles for transfer using the surgical robot are well documented in other sections of this book. However, the concept of dissecting the muscle and then using the robot to place a tension suture in the donor muscle and the suturing the tendon transfer in place has not been previously described. This cadaveric study shows the feasibility of this technique. Current clinical trials are underway to assess long-term clinical results after this procedure.

References

1. Green DP (2005) Radial Nerve Palsy. In: Hotchkiss RN, Pederson WC et al (eds) Green's operative hand surgery. Elsevier Churchill Livingston, Philadelphia
2. House JH (1985) Reconstruction of the thumb in tetraplegia following spinal cord injury. Clin Orthop Relat Res 195:117–128
3. House JH, Gwathmey FW, Lundsgaard DK (1976) Restoration of strong grasp and lateral pinch in the tetraplegic due to cervical spinal cord injury. J Hand Surg 1A:152–159
4. House JH, Shannon MA (1985) Restoration of strong grasp and lateral pinch in tetraplegia: A comparison of two methods of thumb control in each patient. J Hand Surg 10A:22–29
5. House JH, Comadoll J, Dahl AL (1992) One-stage key pinch and release with thumb carpal metacarpal fusion in tetraplegia. J Hand Surg 17A:530–538
6. House JH (1998) Two-stage reconstruction of the tetraplegic hand. In: Walsh TE, Strickland SW (eds) Master techniques in orthopaedic surgery: the hand. Lippincott-Raven, Philadelphia
7. Kozin SH, Bednar M (2001) In vivo determination of available brachioradialis excursion during tetraplegia reconstruction. J Hand Surg 26A:510–514
8. Lieber RL, Murray WM, Clark DL et al (2005) Biomechanical properties of the brachioradialis muscle: Implications for surgical tendon transfer. J Hand Surg 30A:273–282
9. Smeulders MJC, Kreulen MJ, Hage J et al (2002) Progressive surgical dissection for tendon transposition affects length-force characteristics of rat flexor carpi ulnaris muscle. J Orthop Res 20:863–868

Part IV

Clinical Applications

Nerve Entrapment 13

Jose Carlos Garcia Jr.

13.1 Introduction

One of the main advantages of using the surgical robot is minimizing surgical scar. During nerve entrapment releases, one of the tenets of successful surgery is to maintain the nerve in an unscarred bed to prevent postoperative adhesions. However, in many neurolysis procedures, large incisions are placed directly over the site of the nerve. This chapter reviews basic principles of nerve entrapment releases and then demonstrates the advantage of neurolysis with endoscopic and robotic procedures.

Open surgical treatment is the gold standard for peripheral nerve entrapment when conservative treatment is no longer effective. If at surgical exploration the nerve appears intact but compressed by scar, neurolysis is indicated. If a neuroma in continuity is present and a nerve action potential does not conduct along this segment [10], resection of the neuroma and primary grafting should be considered. If a transection or rupture of the nerve is discovered, primary reapproximation and nerve grafting are options.

The procedure should be adapted to the location of the entrapment. For musculocutaneous nerve entrapment, neurolysis is accompanied by an excision of a triangular wedge of the biceps tendon overlying the nerve. Posterior exploration of the quadrilateral space and release of scar or fibrous bands will decompress the axillary nerve [1, 3]. For the suprascapular nerve, an open approach to release of the structures that compress the nerve is technically difficult [14].

The surgical treatment of the thoracic outlet syndrome depends on the structures involved in the pathology. Resection of cervical rib, clavicular osteotomies and

J.C. Garcia Jr., M.D.
Division of Shoulder and Elbow Surgery, NAEON-Center for Advanced Studies in Orthopedics and Neurosurgery, Avenida Macuco 726 cj 1606, São Paulo 04523-001-SP, Brazil
e-mail: josecarlos@especialistadoombro.com.br

P. Liverneaux et al. (eds.), *Telemicrosurgery*,
DOI 10.1007/978-2-8178-0391-3_13, © Springer-Verlag France 2013

osteosynthesis for fractures or fracture sequelae, release of the pectoralis minor, scalenectomy, and simple release are all surgical options. Excellent and good results have been achieved in around 86 % of these surgical procedures [7]. The nerve release may be performed to remove scar tissue and neuromas for spinal accessory nerve entrapment and grafting may be necessary. The dorsal scapular nerve may need scalenectomy of the scalenus medius and neurolysis in order to be decompressed. Surgical options are available for treating injury to the long thoracic nerve in the early stages. Some have favored neurolysis of the nerve with decompression at the level of the scalenus medius or scalenectomy [2]. Other strategies are to perform neurotization (or nerve transfer) using one or two intercostal nerves or the thoracodorsal nerve. In late cases, muscle transfer and scapula-thoracic fusion should be considered [9, 12, 15].

For the radial nerve, attention is directed to releasing compression of the nerve at its division between the posterior interosseous and dorsal sensory branch of the radial nerve as well as at the arcade of Frohse, where the posterior interosseous nerve divides into branches. For Wartenberg syndrome, the fascia between the brachioradialis and extensor carpi radialis longus is released to free the radial sensory nerve from distal to proximal. For the ulnar nerve, the surgical options are neurolysis alone, neurolysis and anterior translocation of the ulnar nerve (subcutaneous or submuscular), or neurolysis and epicondylectomy. For the median nerve, the release of the ligament of Struthers and supracondyloid process, lacertus fibrosus, fascia of the flexor digitorum superficialis muscle, pronator teres, carpal tunnel, or anomalous structures are all surgical options.

13.2 Endoscopic Treatment

Endoscopic treatment for nerve release has been used successfully in many nerve entrapment syndromes such as the carpal tunnel, cubital tunnel, and suprascapular nerve compression. The suprascapular nerve release (Fig. 13.1) has a high rate of successful outcomes but demands a high level of arthroscopic/endoscopic expertise [4, 11]. The carpal tunnel endoscopic release is easy, fast, and presents the advantages of a minimally invasive procedure [13]. Endoscopic release of the ulnar nerve requires advanced endoscopic skills and the surgeon must believe that anterior translocation is unnecessary [8].

Cadaveric studies have also reported of brachial plexus endoscopic exploration. In vivo endoscopic decompression for pectoralis minor syndrome (Fig. 13.2) and anterior axillary nerve release (Fig. 13.3) has been reported.

The advantage of endoscopic procedures is release of large segments of the nerve through small incisions. A major limitation of endoscopic treatment is the two-dimensional view due to the absence of depth perception. The instruments are also limited, lacking three degrees of freedom in order to better access some nerve entrapments sites. Future improvement of endoscopic devices may expand indications for endoscopic release of nerve entrapment.

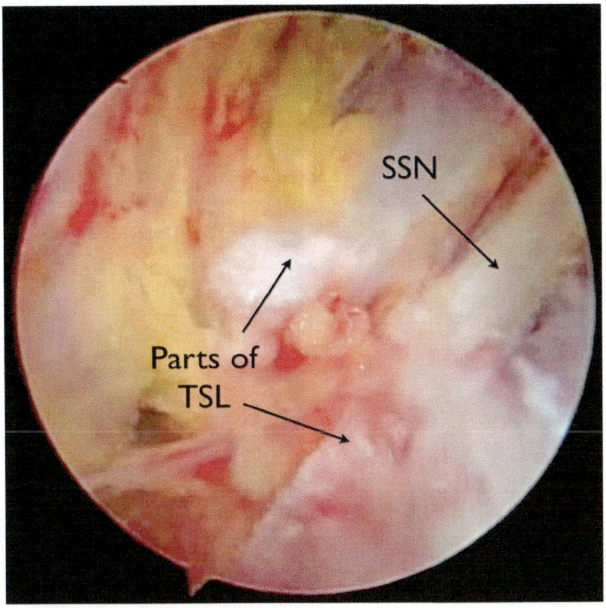

Fig. 13.1 Suprascapular endoscopic release (*SSN* suprascapular nerve, *TSL* transverse superior ligament)

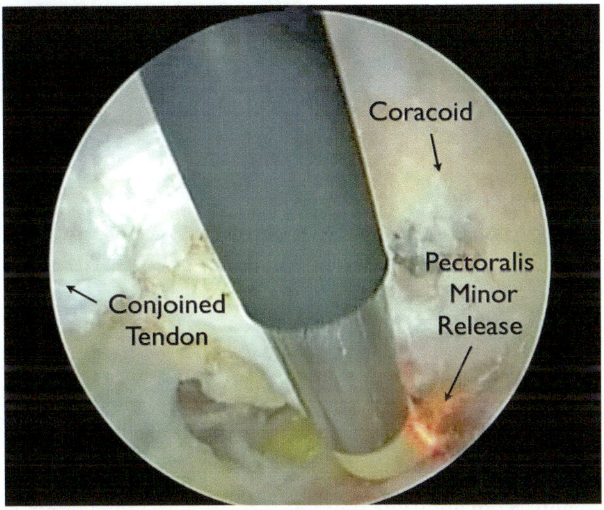

Fig. 13.2 Pectoralis minor detachment from the coracoids

13.3 Robotic-Assisted Treatment

The techniques focusing endorobotic (robotic endoscopy) surgery are still in development in cadaveric models. For thoracic outlet syndrome, anesthetic block landmarks have been used in order to establish the portals. The first supraclavicular portal was made at the lateral border of the sternocleidomastoid muscle, approxi-

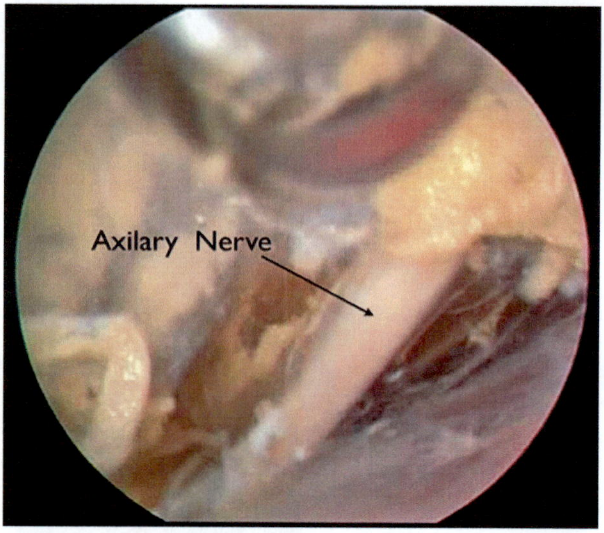

Fig. 13.3 Axillary nerve endoscopic release

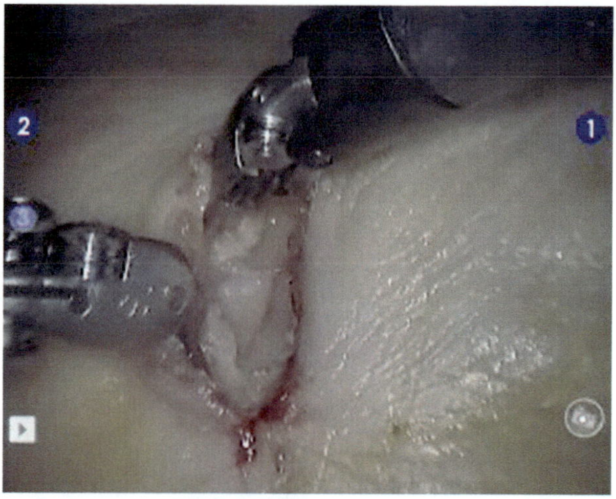

Fig. 13.4 Carpal tunnel release (Courtesy of Philippe Liverneaux)

mately 5 cm above its point of insertion on the clavicle and the second one just above the middle of the clavicle. For other procedures, we are still studying the best choice for portal locations. Some endorobotic procedures, such as suprascapular nerve release, require new tools and different optical angles (30º and 70º) in order to be feasible. Some procedures, such as the carpal tunnel syndrome are already feasible (Fig. 13.4) [6], but the open and endoscopic techniques are faster and cheaper.

At this time, for some procedures in surgical patients, we are doing open robotic surgery, in which we follow the same steps as conventional open surgery mentioned above but use the robot instead of conventional instruments (Figs. 13.5).

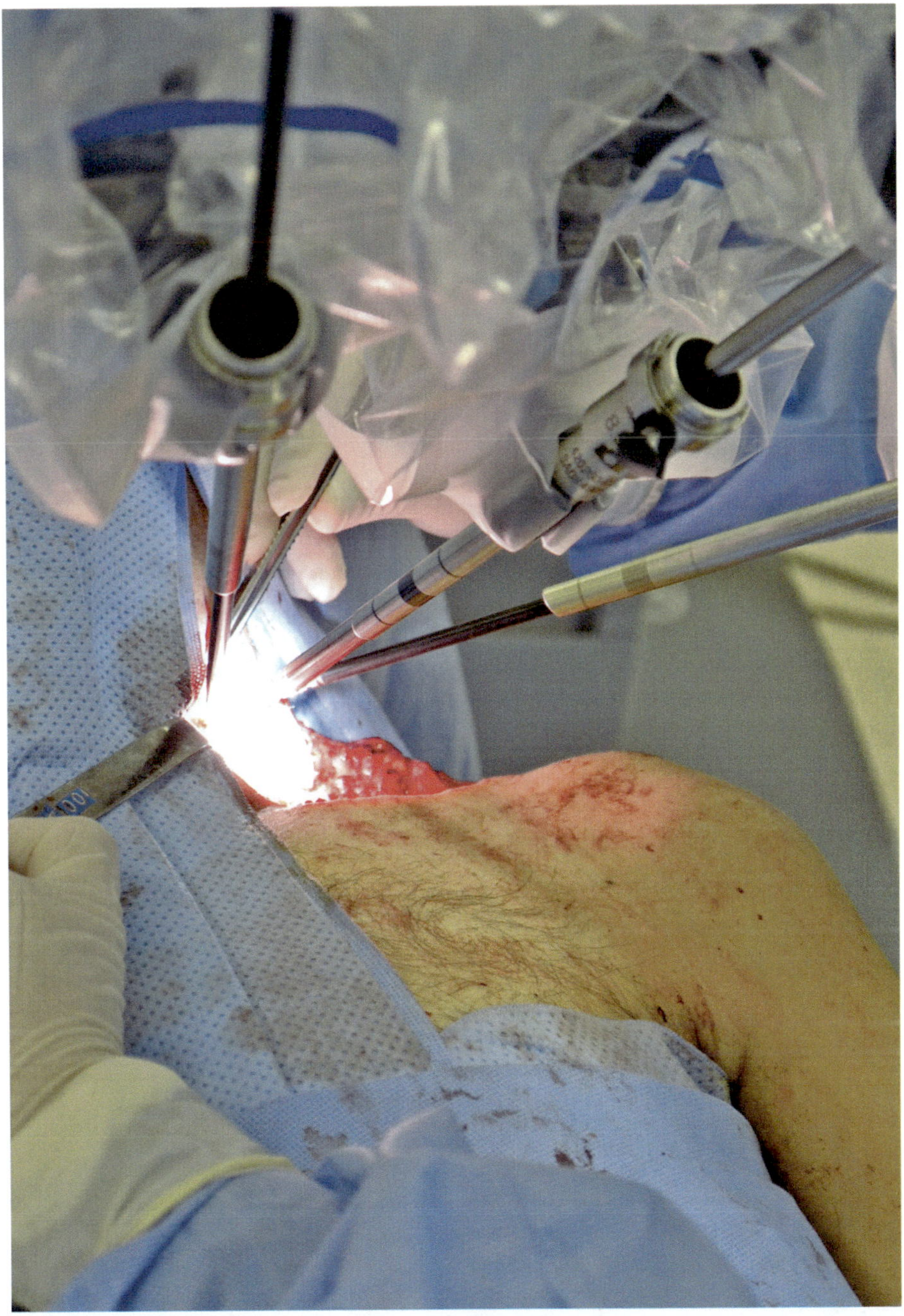

Fig. 13.5 Installation for robotic scalenectomy and brachial plexus release

The release and anterior translocation of the ulnar nerve are already possible by endorobotic surgery (Figs. 13.6–13.8) . To make the ulnar nerve procedures by endorobotic surgery one will need to create a cavity through the portal of the optic, since there are no natural cavities to access the ulnar nerve. The optic's portal is located in the middle third of the arm just above the nerve's path, the other 2 portals are for the robotic arms. They are located 1 to 3 cm distal of the first portal, one medial and the other lateral (Fig. 13.9). A needle can be used to certify the best location of these 2 portals [5].

Robotic-assisted surgery allows for the performance of high dexterity operations with the help of robotic arms and improves technique due to tremor filtration, motion scaling, and ergonomics. The surgeon actually performs a better, more precise, and more highly controlled surgical procedure under high magnification, which may result in an optimal surgical outcome. Other advantages are asepsia instead of antisepsia, with protection of the patient and the surgeon from possible accidents that can spread contagious diseases.

Options for augmented reality also exist. In the future, while the surgeon is performing the surgery, he may simultaneously be able to access 3D patient exams, consult a colleague who is also using a robot online, and browse the Internet for further information. Submicron in vivo histology with real-time functional imaging and diagnosis may help the surgeon in making decision for compressive syndromes secondary to tumors and rheumatic diseases. Specific antibodies and fluorescing markers will be helpful for recognizing structures to access and structures to avoid.

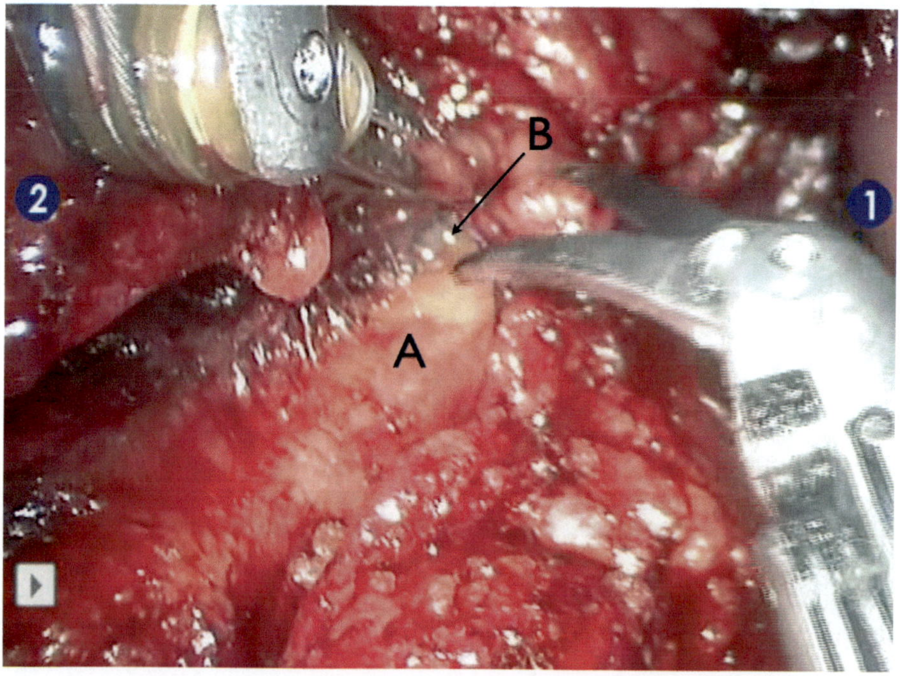

Fig. 13.6 Ulnar nerve endoscopic release. (**a**) Ulnar Nerve (**b**) Cubital Tunnel

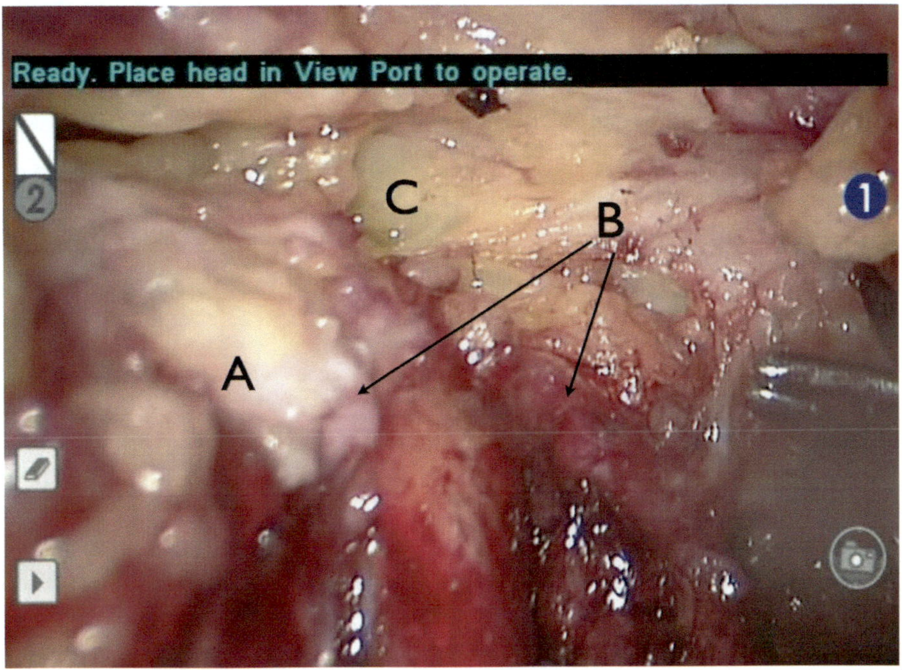

Fig. 13.7 Ulnar nerve endoscopic release. (**a**) Medial epicondyle of the humerus (**b**) Cubital tunnel released (**c**) Osbourn arcade

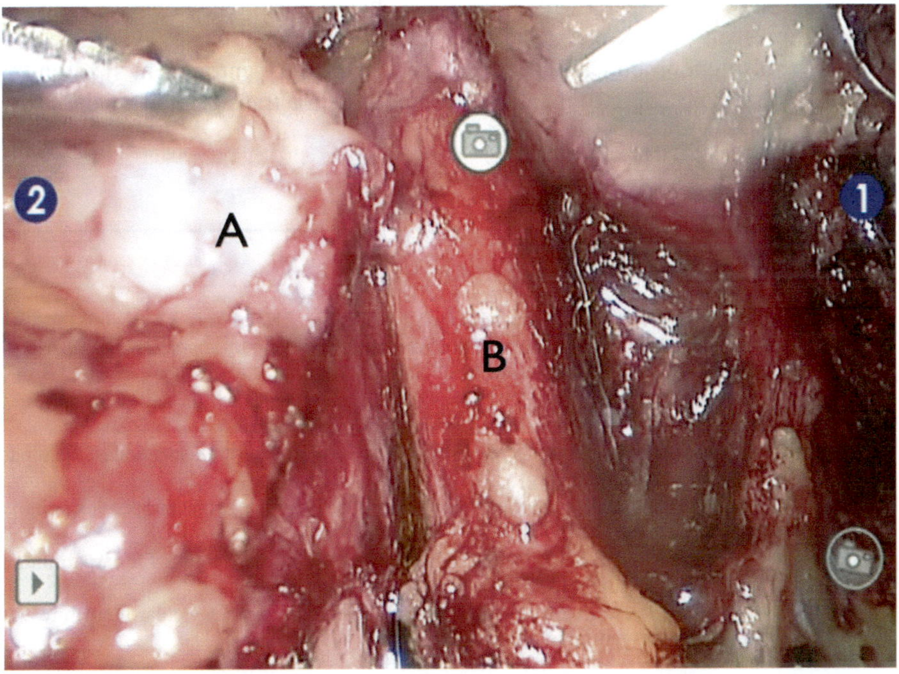

Fig. 13.8 Ulnar nerve endoscopic release. (**a**) Medial epicondyle of the humerus (**b**) Ulnar released

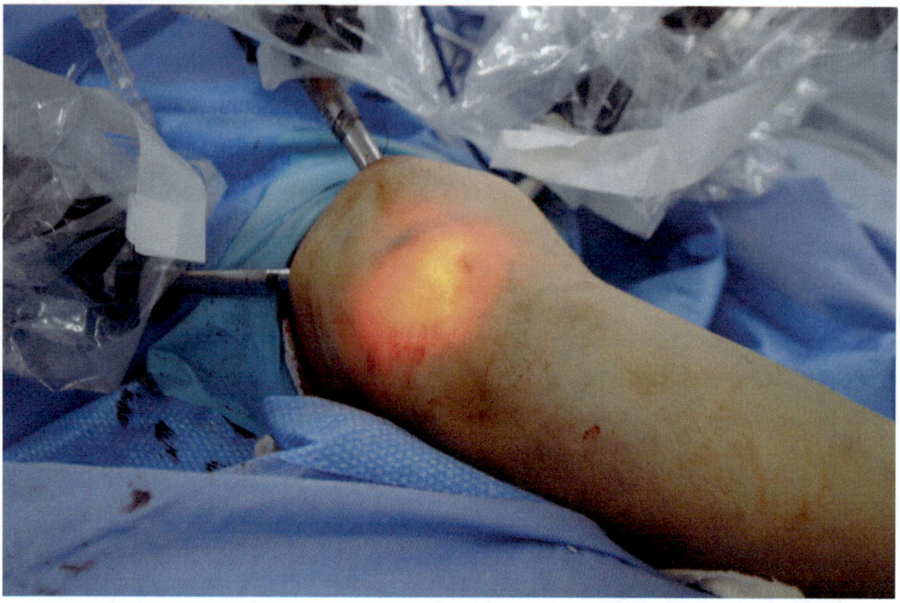

Fig. 13.9 Ulnar nerve endoscopic release in the elbow, external view

Conclusion

In the future, the surgeon will certainly be able to treat brachial plexus injuries, decompress thoracic outlet syndrome, release the teres pronator syndrome and may be also endorobotically access all the other nerve entrapment syndromes. The endorobotic cubital tunnel release and anterior translocation of the ulnar nerve are already in use by the author.

References

1. Cahill BR, Palmer RE (1983) Quadrilateral space syndrome. J Hand Surg 8A:65–69
2. Disa JJ, Wang B, Dellon AL (2001) Correction of scapular winging by supraclavicular neurolysis of the long thoracic nerve. J Reconstr Microsurg 17:79–84
3. Francel TJ, Dellon AL, Campbell JN (1991) Quadrilateral space syndrome: diagnosis and operative decompression technique. Plast Reconstr Surg 87:911–916
4. Garcia JC, Mantovani G, Gouzou S et al (2011) Telerobotic anterior translocation of the ulnar nerve. J Robot Surg 5:153–156
5. Garcia JC (2009) Arthroscopic decompression of the suprascapular nerve: surgical technique. Tech Shoulder Elbow Surg 10:157–159
6. Guldmann R, Pourtales MC, Liverneaux P (2010) Is possible to use robots for carpal tunnel release? J Orthop Sci 15:430–433
7. Hempel GK, Shutz WP, Anderson JF et al (1996) Consecutive supraclavicular first rib resections for thoracic outlet syndrome. Ann Vasc Surg 10:456–462

8. Hoffmann R, Siemionow M (2006) The endoscopic management of cubital tunnel syndrome. J Hand Surg 31B:23–29
9. Jeon IH, Neumann L, Wallace WA (2005) Scapulothoracic fusion for painful winging of the scapula in nondystrophic patients. J Shoulder Elbow Surg 14:400–406
10. Kline DG (2008) Nerve action potential. In: Kline DG, Hudson AR (eds) Nerve injuries: operative results for major nerve injuries, entrapments and tumors, 2nd edn. WB Saunders, Philadelphia, p 83
11. Lafosse L, Piper K, Lanz U (2011) Arthroscopic suprascapular nerve release: indications and technique. J Shoulder Elbow Surg 20:S9–S13
12. Novak CB, Mackinnon SE (2002) Surgical treatment of a long thoracic nerve palsy. Ann Thorac Surg 73:1643–1645
13. Okutsu I, Ninomiya S, Takatori Y et al (1989) Endoscopic management of carpal tunnel syndrome. Arthroscopy 5:11–18
14. Post M, Grinblat E (1993) Suprascapular nerve entrapment: diagnosis and results of treatment. J Shoulder Elbow Surg 2:190–197
15. Povacz P, Resch H (2000) Dynamic stabilization of winging scapula by direct split pectoralis major transfer: a technical note. J Shoulder Elbow Surg 9:76–78

Nerve Repair

14

Stacey H. Berner

14.1 Introduction

During the period between seventh and seventeenth centuries, Paulus Aeginatus, Avicenna, Roger of Salerno, Guglielmo da Saliceto, Guido Lanfranchi, and Gabriele Ferrara, who are universally accepted as the pioneers in this field, introduced the notion of nerve repair [2, 3]. Gabriele Ferrara was the first to give a lucid and succinct description of suturing of the stumps of a transected nerve [1]. Our understanding of nerve injury, repair, and regeneration advanced dramatically over the past century. Military conflicts exposed a great many individuals to penetrating trauma. As battle field resuscitation skills improved, survival rates increased. This provided an opportunity to enhance the understanding of nerve injury and regeneration. The pioneering works of Seddon and Sunderland were based, in large part, on their observations of nerve injuries during and after World War II [6, 7].

Meticulous, tension-free repair is critical to successful nerve repair. This has historically been performed with epineural, fascicular, or epineural perineural repair, and if necessary, grafting of defects [4, 5]. More recently, synthetic conduits, autologous conduits, and acellular allografts have been utilized [4, 8, 9]. Regardless of method of repair, adequate visualization, magnification, and instrumentation are required.

14.1.1 Robot-Assisted Nerve Repair

The principles of nerve repair can be readily carried out with the surgical robot. The precision of gesture associated with the robotic arms make the device ideal for delicate, microneural repair. Although the clinical experience to date is small, it is growing. Similar to traditional repair, primary neurorrhaphy of nerve lacerations can be performed

S.H. Berner, M.D.
Department of Orthopedic Surgery, Northwest Hospital,
10 Crossroads Drive, Suite 210, Owings Mills, Baltimore, MD, USA
e-mail: sberner@surgcenter.com

P. Liverneaux et al. (eds.), *Telemicrosurgery*,
DOI 10.1007/978-2-8178-0391-3_14, © Springer-Verlag France 2013

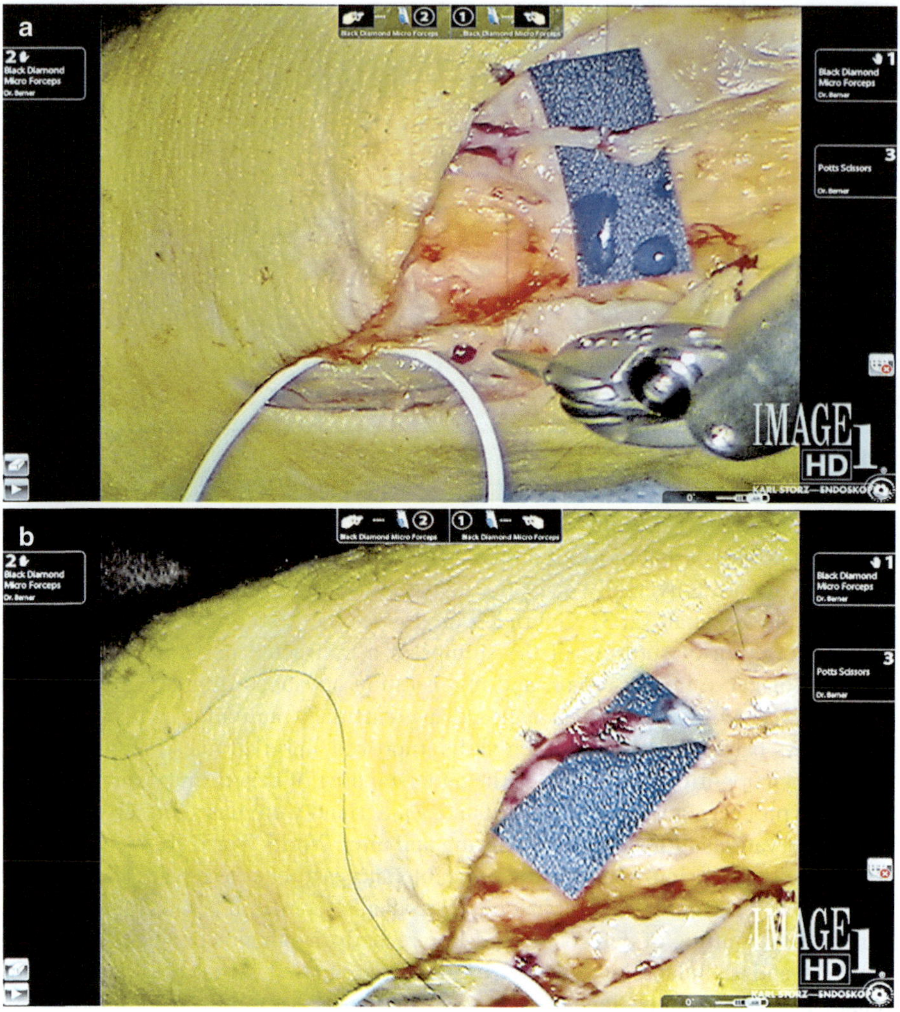

Fig. 14.1 Radial nerve injury. (**a**) Superficial radial nerve laceration. (**b**) Superficial radial nerve repair

with epineural repair (Fig. 14.1). For those injuries with significant loss of nerve structure, or extensive nerve damage, primary or secondary grafting procedures can be performed (Fig. 14.2). Neural conduits can be easily manipulated and sutured with the robot when the surgeon encounters cases on nerve injury with modest gaps that cannot be overcome by mobilization of the nerve ends (Fig. 14.3).

As the surgeon's familiarity with robotically assisted primary and secondary repair increases, it is likely that additional benefits of this new technology will be realized. Future robotic endeavors will likely include ultrahigh magnification or so-called super microsurgery. Advanced staining and mapping techniques may improve the ability to create a perfect match of motor and sensory fascicles when repairing mixed nerve

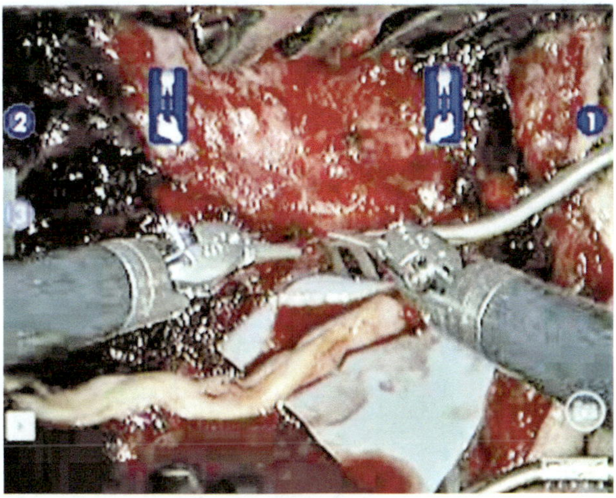

Fig. 14.2 Radial nerve graft (Courtesy of Philippe Liverneaux)

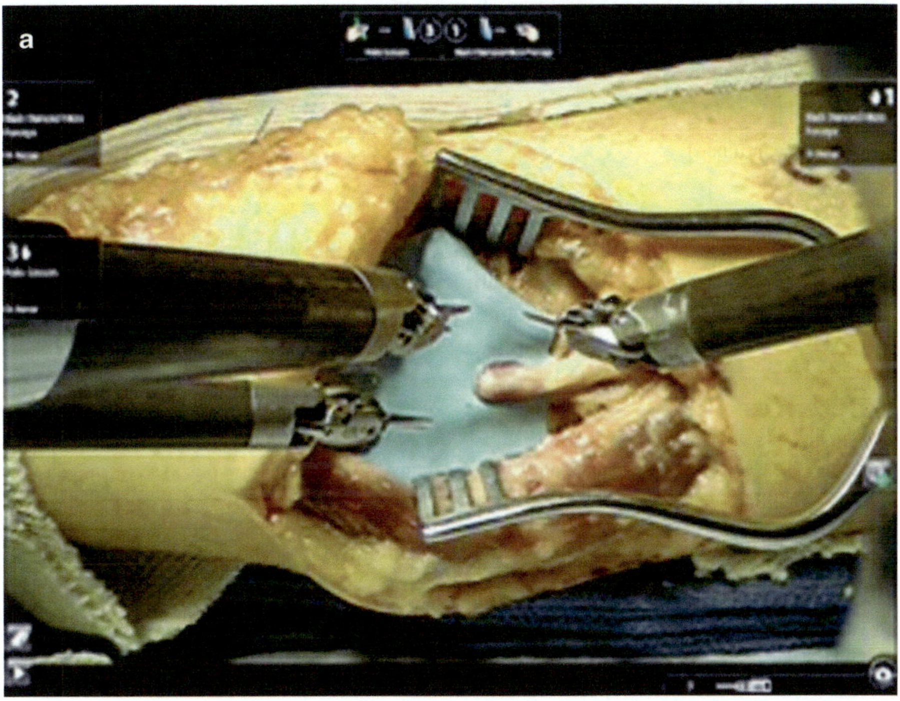

Fig. 14.3 Ulnar nerve. (**a**) Subacute ulnar nerve laceration on distal forearm. (**b**) Ulnar nerve repair with neural conduit

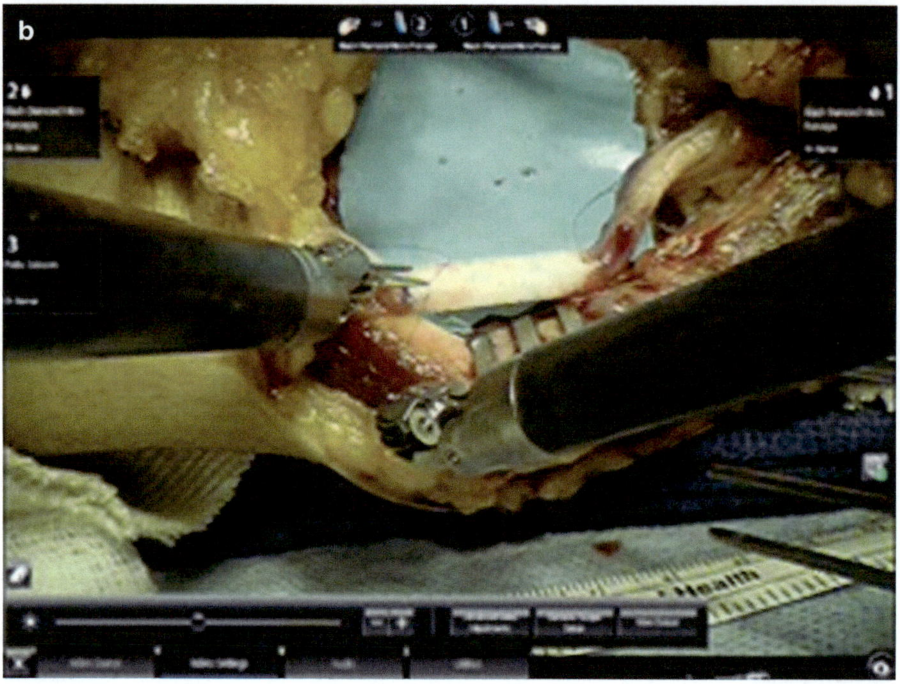

Fig. 14.3 (continued)

injuries. New techniques of nerve coaptation or tissue welding will likely facilitate anastomosing extremely tiny and complex neural structures with great precision. Hopefully, this will lead to enhanced nerve recovery and regeneration.

References

1. Artico M, Cervoni L, Nucci F et al (1996) Birthday of peripheral nervous system surgery: the contribution of Gabriele Ferrara (1543–1627). Neurosurgery 39:380–382
2. Belen D, Aciduman A, Er U (2009) History of peripheral nerve repair: may the procedure have been practiced in Hippocratic school? Surg Neurol 72:190–193
3. Bora FW Jr, Pleasurable DE, Didizian NA (1976) A study of nerve regeneration and neuroma formation after nerve suture by various techniques. J Hand Surg 1A:138–143
4. Bora FW Jr, Bednar JM, Osterman AL et al (1987) Prosthetic nerve grafts: a resorbable tube as an alternative to autogenous nerve grafting. J Hand Surg 12A:685–692
5. Cabaud HE, Rodkey WG, McCarroll HR et al (1976) Epineural and perineural fascicular nerve repairs: a critical comparison. J Hand Surg 1A:131–137
6. Seddon HJ (1972) Disorders of the peripheral nerves. William and Wilkins, Baltimore
7. Sunderland S (1978) Nerves and nerve injuries, 2nd edn. Churchill Livingstone, New York
8. Weber RA, Breidenbach WC, Brown R et al (2000) Randomized prospective study of polyglycolic acid conduits for digital nerve reconstruction in humans. Plas Reconstr Surg 106:1036–1045
9. Whitlock E, Tuffaha S, Luciano JP et al (2009) Processed allografts and type I collagen conduits for repair of peripheral nerve gaps. Muscle Nerve 39:787–799

Brachial Plexus

15

Kiyohito Naito, Mickaël Ohana, Thierry Lequint, Sybille Facca, and Philippe Liverneaux

15.1 Introduction

Minimally invasive surgery has quickly become the first therapeutic option in many operative indications, reducing postoperative complications and increasing patient comfort. Surgical robotics already proved useful, leading to numerous enhancements of the technique [1, 2].

Several interventions remain almost inaccessible to endoscopic surgery, such as brachial plexus injuries, affecting mostly young patients and leading to severe functional disability [3]. Open techniques are still the gold standard of brachial plexus surgery [4]. Development of minimally invasive and robot-assisted surgical approaches has the potential to greatly improve the surgical outcome.

K. Naito, M.D.
Department of Hand Surgery, Strasbourg University Hospital,
10 Avenue Baumann, F-67403 Illkirch, Strasbourg, France

Department of Orthopeadics, Juntendo University, Tokyo, Japan

M. Ohana, M.D.
Department of Radiology, Strasbourg University Hospital, Strasbourg, France

T. Lequint, M.D.
Department of Hand Surgery, Strasbourg University Hospital,
10 Avenue Baumann, F-67403 Illkirch, Strasbourg, France

Department of Orthopeadics, Grand Hôpital, Charleroi, Belgium

S. Facca, M.D.
Department of Hand Surgery, Strasbourg University Hospital,
10 Avenue Baumann, F-67403 Illkirch, Strasbourg, France

P. Liverneaux, M.D., Ph.D. (✉)
Department of Hand Surgery, Strasbourg University Hospital,
10 Avenue Baumann, F-67403 Illkirch, Strasbourg, France

European Institute of TeleSurgery, IRCAD, F-67000 Strasbourg, France
e-mail: philippe.liverneaux@chru-strasbourg.fr

P. Liverneaux et al. (eds.), *Telemicrosurgery*,
DOI 10.1007/978-2-8178-0391-3_15, © Springer-Verlag France 2013

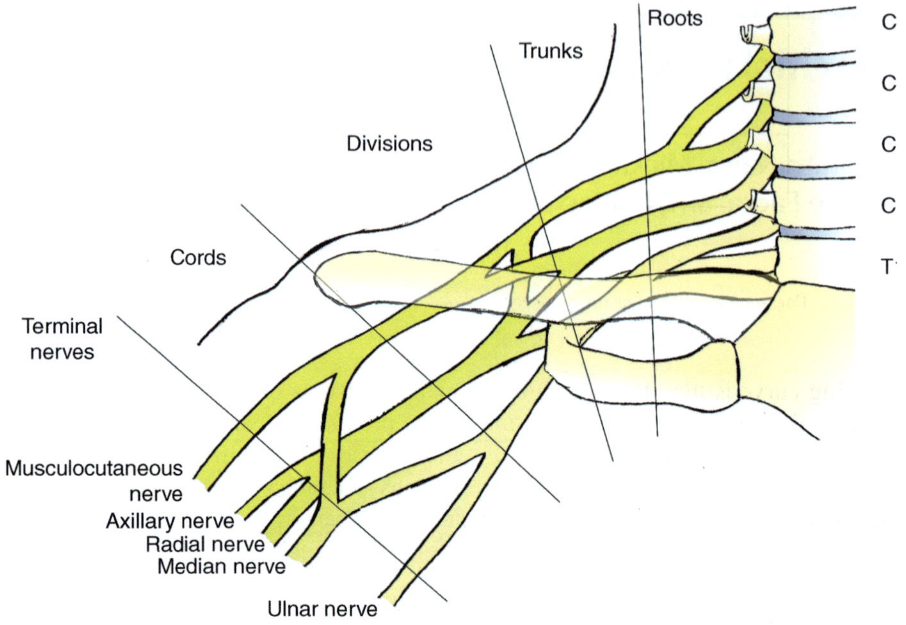

Fig. 15.1 Schematic normal anatomy of the brachial plexus (Drawing courtesy of Dr W. Ohana)

15.2 Current Management of Brachial Plexus Injuries

15.2.1 Anatomy

Brachial plexus (Fig. 15.1) is formed by the confluence of the ventral rami of the spinal nerve roots from C5 to T1 [5] and provides the sensory-motor innervation of the upper limb.

In its modal distribution (about 40 % of cases), the five ventral rami of the spinal nerve roots merge into three trunks, each one splitting into a posterior and anterior division. These divisions anastomose each other to form the three cords of the brachial plexus, from which detach the terminal branches (musculocutaneous nerve, axillary nerve, ulnar nerve, radial nerve, and median nerve).

There are substantial variations in this anatomy, both among different subjects and between the left and the right side of a same individual [5, 6]. Most common variants involve the participation of the C4 root (prefixed plexus) or the T2 root (postfixed plexus). This variability partly accounts for the difficulties of the surgery.

15.2.2 Etiologies and Classification of Brachial Plexus Injuries

The vast majority of brachial plexus injuries are traumatic, resulting from traction of the nerves during violent elongation movements. These injuries occur commonly after motorcycle accident [7] or shoulder dislocation [8]. They can also be of iatrogenic origin, with lesions by positional stretching of the brachial plexus occurring after long interventions [9, 10] or interventional radiology procedures [11], or by direct section of the nerve during cervical surgery [12].

Distinction is made between pre- and postganglionic lesions.

Preganglionic lesions correspond to the avulsion of the dorsal or ventral rootlets at the spinal cord. They usually lead to the formation of a pseudomeningocele [13].

Postganglionic lesions are related either with a nerve crush or a rupture of continuity in a nerve branch [6]. These lesions are best described using Seddon's classification, refined by Sunderland [14], and based on the nerve fiber histology. Thus, the higher the nerve ultrastructure is disrupted, the less the spontaneous nerve regeneration is likely to occur.

In 15 % of cases, posttraumatic lesions are both pre- and postganglionic [15].

Non-traumatic lesions of the brachial plexus are less common [16]: Parsonage-Turner syndrome, primary tumors of neurogenic (neurinomas, neurofibromas, neurofibrosarcomas) or non-neurogenic origin (hamartoma, desmoid tumor), tumoral infiltration (Pancoast-Tobias syndrome, seen in apical lung carcinoma), postradiation plexopathy, post-infectious neuropathies [17] and thoracic outlet syndrome [18, 19].

15.2.3 Therapeutic

The diagnosis of brachial plexus injuries is primarily clinical, by comparative exploration of muscular and sensitive territories. A classification of the type of nerve lesion can be obtained in most cases by correlation with medical history and electromyogram results.

Imaging can provide useful additional information. In emergency situations, it can assess associated injuries: plain radiographs and CT angiography represent the best modalities for evaluation of associated bone and vascular lesions. In more chronic conditions or in the monitoring of stretching/compression lesions, MRI is the first-line exam [20], allowing accurate determination of pre- and postganglionic injuries (Figs. 15.2 and 15.3) as well as exploration of cervical spinal cord and perineural space.

The management of brachial plexus injuries is not fully codified and is subject to variations depending on the teams and centers involved [4, 6, 15, 21–26].

Neurological deficits following penetrating trauma should benefit from immediate surgical exploration (<72 h), in an attempt of nerve reparation, either by direct nerve suture or autologous nerve graft.

Stretch or blunt injuries may correspond to a lower degree lesion in the Sunderland classification, with a good chance of spontaneous recovery. Therapeutic attitude is thus a "wait and see" approach. In the absence of clinical recovery and after MRI and EMG examinations, surgical exploration is performed within 3–6 months after initial injury and includes neurolysis (freeing the nerve from its adhesions) and a determination of the lesional grade. If a high-degree lesion is confirmed, a direct nerve suture or, more often, an autologous nerve graft is performed.

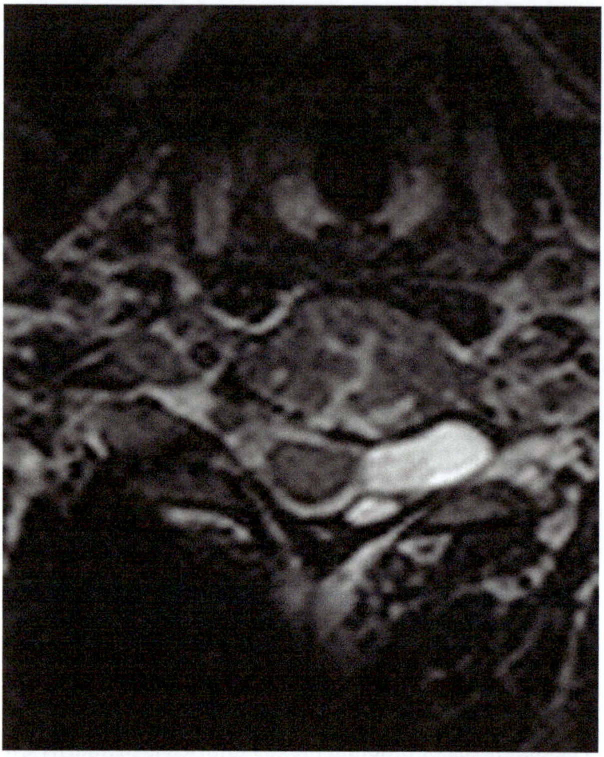

Fig. 15.2 Cervical spine MRI; axial T2-weighted slice. Pseudomeningocele at the level of C7 left rootlets: preganglionic avulsion after a motorcycle accident

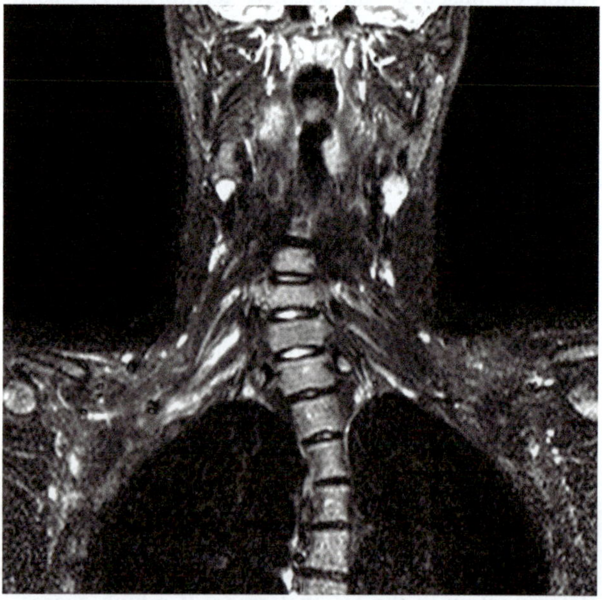

Fig. 15.3 Brachial plexus MRI; coronal STIR slice. Global hypersignal and thickening of the cords of the right brachial plexus: posttraumatic postganglionic injury (axonotmesis) after a direct trauma

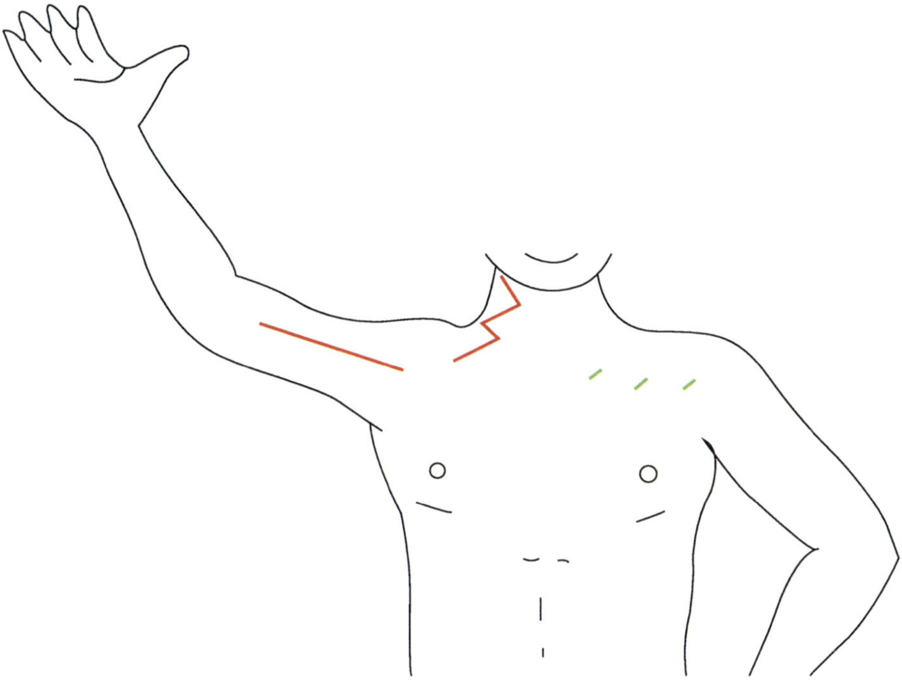

Fig. 15.4 *Red lines*: conventional approach for open surgery of the brachial plexus. Extensive dissection leading to superficial and internal scars. *Green spots*: mini-invasive approach

15.2.4 Problematic

All these techniques are currently open procedures, thus requiring large incisions, from the mastoid to the upper third of the arm (Fig. 15.4). In addition to an obvious aesthetic prejudice in often-young patients, internal scars may induce perineural sclerosis and interfere with axonal regeneration. Minimally invasive surgery could significantly reduce these issues.

15.3 Minimally Invasive Robot-Assisted Brachial Plexus Surgery

15.3.1 Telemicrosurgery

Da Vinci® (Intuitive Surgical™, Sunnyvale, CA) is the most widely used surgical robot [27–29]; it is also the only one to be commercially available. It is a master/slave system, consisting of a remote terminal with joysticks and high-resolution 3D screens, and a patient end made of three to four robotic arms and proprietary instruments (Fig. 15.5).

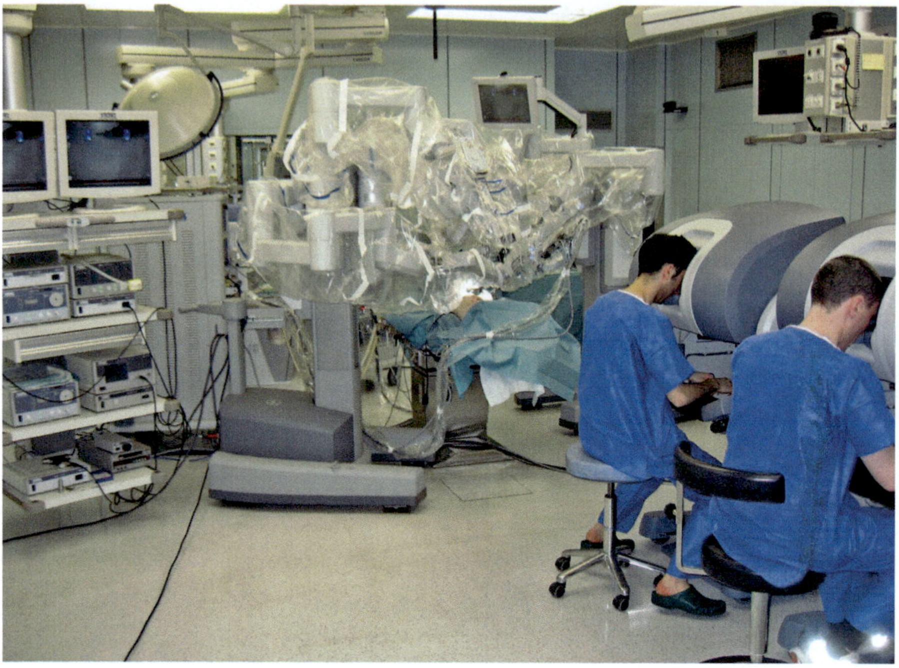

Fig. 15.5 Da Vinci robotic system as used in telemicrosurgery

The advantages of a telemanipulator are numerous: suppression of physiological tremor, optical magnification of the surgeon's movements, and improved ergonomics of the console [30] and augmented reality guidance and learning using a virtual patient model.

All these features contribute to an improvement of the surgical technique, leading to a sharp increase in the surgeon's accuracy.

In microsurgery, these benefits are therefore particularly useful, and telesurgery allows a greater efficiency in peripheral nerve repair [31]. We were able to prove, in many biological models (rats, pigs, and fresh cadavers), the feasibility and the reliability of telemicrosurgery for direct nerve suture and neurotropic repair using a nerve regrowth guide. All the repairs were achieved within a reasonable operating time and with a short learning curve [31].

Among the drawbacks of the technique are, in addition to its high cost, a lack of dedicated microsurgery instrumentation and a force feedback insufficient for providing useful tactile feeling.

15.3.2 Minimally Invasive Approaches

It seems logical to gather telemicrosurgery and minimally invasive surgery to operate in subcutaneous spaces through infracentimetric incisions (concept of tele-

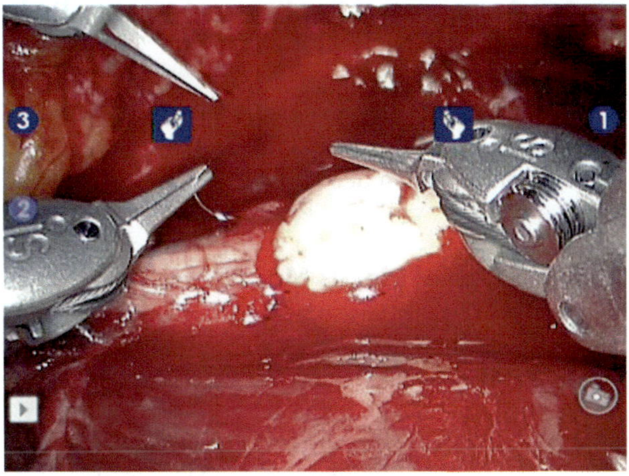

Fig. 15.6 Example of direct nerve suture under telemicrosurgery

endomicrosurgery). Such an approach requires the creation of a central resection cavity, usually done in two steps, one superficial and a second consisting of a deeper dissection to liberate perineural spaces. Maintaining this working chamber requires an insufflation of carbon dioxide and/or the use of specific surgical retractors.

Our clinical experience is based on 12 cases of brachial plexus tele-endomicrosurgery.

Considering the microsurgical gesture, all nerve repairs were achieved under excellent conditions (Fig. 15.6).

Considering the minimally invasive approach, results are yet inconclusive, with a need to convert to open surgery in nine cases. The reasons for conversion were numerous: difficulties to maintain the resection cavity (leakage of carbon dioxide through trocar holes), unsuited instrumentation, blurring of the stereoscopic vision (due to a rapid increase in temperature in this small volume and solved by the use of a suction device), and major difficulties in visual identification of anatomical landmarks.

15.3.3 Problematic

Minimally invasive and robot-assisted surgery of the brachial plexus is possible, though it is still very challenging due to the complexity of the anatomy of this structure.

Development of a dedicated instrumentation should address several pitfalls, such as the difficulty of maintaining carbon dioxide within the working chamber, and the perfect adaptation of the surgical material to the operative field size.

Lack of direct visualization of anatomical landmarks could be addressed by using a peroperative computer aid to track and identify these structures. Augmented reality can respond to this need [32–40].

15.4 Augmented Reality and Minimally Invasive Surgery of the Brachial Plexus

In an augmented reality process, a virtual patient modelized from imaging acts as a guide for the surgeon, providing information registered with operative reality and allowing optimization of surgical approach, incisions, and navigation.

15.4.1 Brachial Plexus Modelization

This is an essential preliminary step, using medical imaging and posttreatment techniques. In the brachial plexus context, CT and MRI are the two modalities of choice.

15.4.1.1 CT Modelization

CT is based on X-ray attenuation [41]. Combined with intravenous injection of contrast (CT angiography), it allows an excellent exploration of both bone and vascular structures, due to its high spatial resolution. 3D acquisition covers a wide field in seconds, with an isotropic voxel, allowing application of many posttreatments and reconstructions.

There are two 3D modelization techniques: volume rendering end segmentation.

Volume rendering is based on density difference and assigns a color and a transparency to each voxel, depending on its density value. In the obtained volume, 3D structures correspond to the summation of different voxels' transparencies (Fig. 15.7).

Segmentation is based on a time-consuming delineation of structures of interest, made manually or semiautomatically. Thus defined, 3D structures are displayed with surface rendering, with a good visual result, and can be hidden or shown at will.

The best result is obtained with volume rendering of CT angiography: vascular and bone reconstruction are of excellent quality and produced quickly and easily. Even though the CT low-contrast resolution does not allow direct visualization of the brachial plexus, information provided is valuable, particularly the clear identification of vertebral foramina which allows to track the emerging nerve roots.

15.4.1.2 MRI Modelization

MRI excellent contrast resolution and good spatial resolution allow simultaneous assessment of the spinal cord, nerve roots, vessel, and soft tissues of the neck. Best results are obtained with a T2-weighted sequence with fat suppression (STIR sequences in particular) [42, 43]. The STIR sequence provides an excellent contrast between the neural structures, which have a hyperintense signal due to their large water content, and the surrounding structures.

Newly developed isotropic 3D sequence [44, 45] enables an advanced post-processing very similar to what is obtained with CT images: multiplanar reconstructions, maximum intensity projection, volume rendering, and surface rendering (Figs. 15.8 and 15.9). However, the similar intensity of bone and muscle makes the

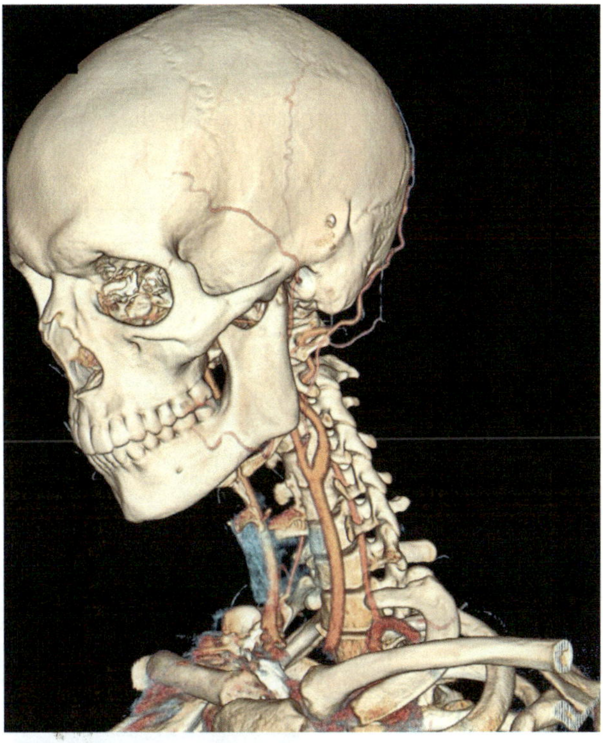

Fig. 15.7 Volume rendering obtained from cervical CT angiography. Excellent visualization of bone and vascular structures

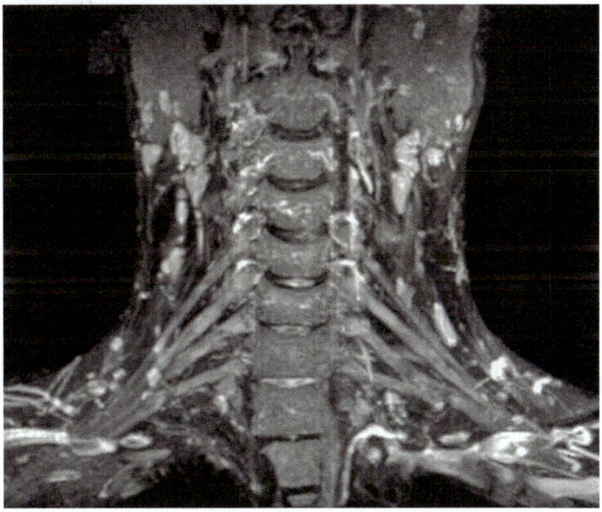

Fig. 15.8 MIP (maximum intensity projection) obtained from a 3D STIR acquisition of a normal brachial plexus. Excellent direct visualization of trunks and cords

volume rendering and the semiautomatic segmentation difficult. Final results are visually thrilling, perfect for a first global approach, but do not offer a sufficient spatial resolution, as permitted by the native millimetric acquisition.

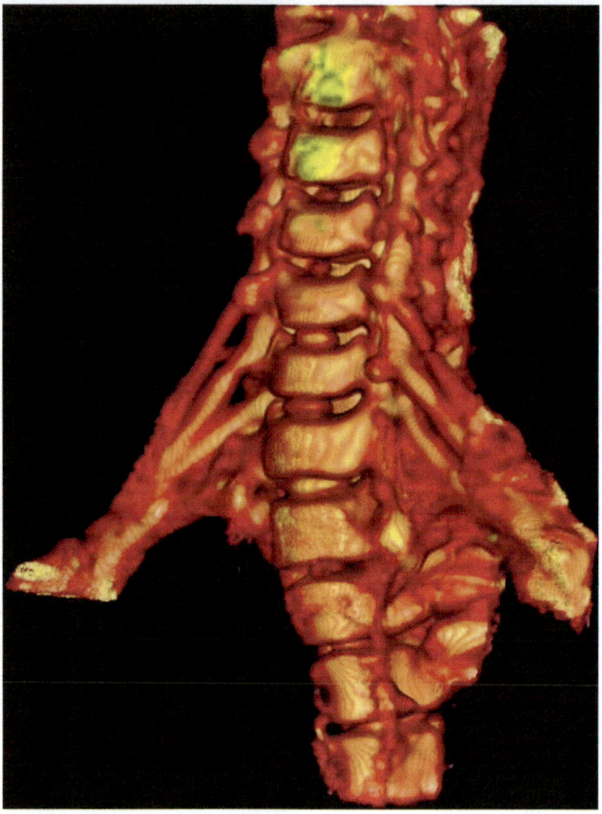

Fig. 15.9 Volume rendering obtained from a 3D STIR acquisition of a normal brachial plexus, after extensive manual post-processing. Good 3D visualization of trunks and vertebral bodies

Functional imaging is a booming imaging field. Tractography is an MRI technique based on diffusion, aiming at the reconstruction of nerve fibers. Its application in brachial plexus modelization is still limited by technological constraints, but preliminary results are very encouraging (Fig. 15.10).

15.4.2 Peroperative Registration

Once patient modelization is performed, registration between the model and surgical reality is yet to be done.

Registration can be rigid (direct application of data) or nonrigid (adaptation of raw data to the surgical reality using mathematical deformation) [39]. Nonrigid registration can be improved in real time with mathematical modelization of deformations induced by surgical instruments or patient movement (especially breathing) [46].

Registration can be interactive (the user adjusts the position of the model with the one of the real patient using internal or external landmarks) or automatic. Registration can be facilitated by the use of additional markers (optical, infrared, electromagnetic [47]) in order to track in real time their position.

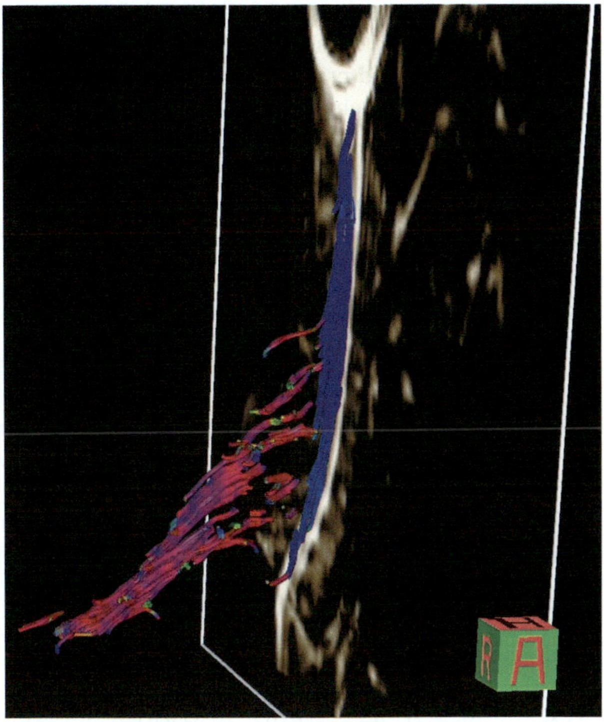

Fig. 15.10 Tractography of a normal right brachial plexus. Nice visualization of trunks and cords

Information is brought to the surgeon through various techniques of augmented reality [37], such as external display, head-up display, or direct projection on the patient's skin.

15.4.3 Augmented Reality Project in Brachial Plexus Surgery

The use of augmented reality could greatly reduce or even completely remove the landmark identification constraints associated with minimally invasive surgery and therefore increase the effectiveness and safety of this surgical approach.

We propose four steps for achieving this goal.

The first one is the fusion between a volume rendering coming from a CT angiography and tractography. This fusion would allow simultaneous 3D visualization of bone, arteries, and nerve roots, providing sufficient information for immediate recognition of all anatomical landmarks by the surgeon [48].

The second is the display of these 3D data within the native 3D STIR volume. Referring to the original sequence could be useful when ultraprecise positioning is needed.

The third is the real-time implementation, within this virtual volume, of the endoscope's position ("virtual endoscope"), thanks to external markers (optical or electromagnetic).

The last one is the display of all these information on an external screen, next to the surgeon's remote console.

This system would provide a 3D default view showing bone structure, arteries, and the roots of the brachial plexus, with real-time implementation of the endoscope's position. This "simplified" view should allow quick identification and endoscope reposition if necessary. Should precise positioning or identification of an anatomical structure not shown in 3D be needed, the ability to switch back to 3D STIR native sequence would be sufficient to compensate the 3D reconstructions' lack of precision.

Conclusion

Contributions of robotics in microsurgery are sharp and clearly demonstrated and justify its use in the surgical repair of peripheral nerves. A minimally invasive approach should result in significant aesthetic and functional benefits.

In brachial plexus surgery, tele-endomicrosurgery is feasible but faces major constraints regarding the creation, maintenance, and navigation inside the working chamber. Adaptation of the endoscopic equipment and use of advanced techniques of augmented reality should address most of these problems.

References

1. Ayav A, Bresler L, Brunaud L, Boissel P (2004) Early results of one-year robotic surgery using the Da Vinci system to perform advanced laparoscopic procedures. J Gastrointest Surg 8(6): 720–726
2. Naito K, Facca S, Lequint T, Liverneaux P (2012) Oberlin's procedure for restoration of elbow flexion with Da Vinci robot: 4 cases. Plast Reconstr Surg 129(3):707–11
3. Novak CB, Anastakis DJ, Beaton DE, Mackinnon SE, Katz J (2010) Relationships among pain disability, pain intensity, illness intrusiveness, and upper extremity disability in patients with traumatic peripheral nerve injury. J Hand Surg 35(10):1633–1639
4. Greenfield BH, Geist K (2011) Evaluation and treatment of brachial plexus lesions. In: Physical therapy of the shoulder, 5th edn. Churchill Livingstone, Saint Louis, pp 163–183
5. Bollini CA, Wikinski JA (2006) Anatomical review of the brachial plexus. Tech Reg Anesth Pain Manag 10(3):69–78
6. Gregory J, Cowey A, Jones M, Pickard S, Ford D (2009) The anatomy, investigations and management of adult brachial plexus injuries. Orthop Trauma 23(6):420–432
7. Altaf F, Mannan K, Sinisi M, Birch R (2008) Severe brachial plexus injuries in rugby: mechanisms and management. Inj Extra 39(5):206–206
8. Kosiyatrakul A, Jitprapaikulsarn S, Durand S, Oberlin C (2009) Recovery of brachial plexus injury after shoulder dislocation. Injury 40(12):1327–1329
9. Shveiky D, Aseff JN, Iglesia CB (2010) Brachial plexus injury after laparoscopic and robotic surgery. J Minim Invasive Gynecol 17(4):414–420
10. Pillai AK, Ferral H, Desai S, Paruchuri S, Asselmeier S, Perez-Gautrin R (2007) Brachial plexus injury related to patient positioning. J Vasc Interv Radiol 18(7):833–834
11. Hiraki T, Gobara H, Mimura H, Sano Y, Toyooka S, Shibamoto K, Kishi R, Uka M, Kanazawa S (2010) Brachial nerve injury caused by percutaneous radiofrequency ablation of apical lung cancer: a report of four cases. J Vasc Interv Radiol 21(7):1129–1133

12. Monteiro MJ, Altman K, Khandwala A (2010) Injury to the brachial plexus in neck dissections. Br J Oral Maxillofac Surg 48(3):197–198
13. Castillo M (2005) Imaging the anatomy of the brachial plexus: review and self-assessment module. AJR Am J Roentgenol 185(6 Suppl):S196–S204
14. Moser T, Kremer S, Holl N (2009) Imagerie du nerf peripherique: anatomie, techniques d'exploration et principales pathologies. J Radiol 90(10):1448–1448
15. Brophy RH, Wolfe SW (2005) Planning brachial plexus surgery: treatment options and priorities. Hand Clin 21(1):47–54
16. Mullins GM, O'Sullivan SS, Neligan A, Daly S, Galvin RJ, Sweeney BJ, McNamara B (2007) Non-traumatic brachial plexopathies, clinical, radiological and neurophysiological findings from a tertiary centre. Clin Neurol Neurosurg 109(8):661–666
17. Choi J-Y, Kang CH, Kim B-J, Park K-W, Yu S-W (2009) Brachial plexopathy following herpes zoster infection: two cases with MRI findings. J Neurol Sci 285(1–2):224–226
18. Hof JJ, Kliot M, Slimp J, Haynor DR (2008) What's new in MRI of peripheral nerve entrapment? Neurosurg Clin N Am 19(4):583–595
19. Cotten A, Chantelot C, Duquesnoy B, Demondion X (2007) Imagerie des syndromes de la traversée cervicothoracobrachiale. Rev Rhum 74(4):333–338
20. Lacour MC (2009) Intérêt de l'imagerie dans le diagnostic des plexopathies. Rev Neurol 165(12):1134–1139
21. Giuffre JL, Kakar S, Bishop AT, Spinner RJ, Shin AY (2010) Current concepts of the treatment of adult brachial plexus injuries. J Hand Surg 35(4):678–688
22. Mannan K, Carlstedt T (2006) Injuries to the brachial plexus. Surgery (Oxford) 24(12): 409–414
23. Parvizi J, Kim GK (2010) Brachial plexus injury. High Yield Orthopaedics. W.B. Saunders, Philadelphia, In, pp 68–69
24. Shenaq SM, Kim JYS, Bullocks J, Joseph GM, Robert DG, Sean GB (2006) Brachial plexus injuries. In: Current therapy in plastic surgery. W.B. Saunders, Philadelphia, pp 574–583
25. Thornton DJA, Kay SPJ (2010) A clinical approach to the management of brachial plexus and peripheral nerve injury. Surgery (Oxford) 28(2):79–84
26. Liverneaux PA, Diaz LC, Beaulieu J-Y, Durand S, Oberlin C (2006) Preliminary results of double nerve transfer to restore elbow flexion in upper type brachial plexus palsies. Plast Reconstr Surg 117(3):915–9
27. Moten SC, Kypson AP, Chitwood WR Jr, Joseph AS Jr, Ashutosh T (2008) Use of robotics in other surgical specialties. In: Robotics in urologic surgery. W.B. Saunders, Philadelphia, pp 159–173
28. Zacharopoulou C, Sananes N, Baulon E, Garbin O, Wattiez A (2010) Chirurgie robotique en gynécologie: état des connaissances. Revue de la littérature. J Gynecol Obstet Biol Reprod 39(6):444–452
29. Kim HL, Schulam P (2004) The PAKY, HERMES, AESOP, ZEUS, and da Vinci robotic systems. Urol Clin North Am 31(4):659–669
30. Byrn JC, Schluender S, Divino CM, Conrad J, Gurland B, Shlasko E, Szold A (2007) Three-dimensional imaging improves surgical performance for both novice and experienced operators using the da Vinci Robot System. Am J Surg 193(4):519–522
31. Nectoux E, Taleb C, Liverneaux P (2009) Nerve repair in telemicrosurgery: an experimental study. J Reconstr Microsurg 25(4):261–265
32. Marescaux J, Soler L, Rubino F (2005) Augmented reality for surgery and interventional therapy. Oper Tech Gen Surg 7(4):182–187
33. Nicolau SA, Pennec X, Soler L, Buy X, Gangi A, Ayache N, Marescaux J (2009) An augmented reality system for liver thermal ablation: design and evaluation on clinical cases. Med Image Anal 13(3):494–506
34. Freudenthal A, Stüdeli T, Lamata P, Samset E (2010) Collaborative co-design of emerging multi-technologies for surgery. J Biomed Inform 44(2):198–215

35. Lee S-L, Lerotic M, Vitiello V, Giannarou S, Kwok K-W, Visentini-Scarzanella M, Yang G-Z (2010) From medical images to minimally invasive intervention: computer assistance for robotic surgery. Comput Med Imaging Graph 34(1):33–45
36. Teber D, Guven S, Simpfendörfer T, Baumhauer M, Güven EO, Yencilek F, Gözen AS, Rassweiler J (2009) Augmented reality: a new tool to improve surgical accuracy during laparoscopic partial nephrectomy? Preliminary in vitro and in vivo results. Eur Urol 56(2):332–338
37. Ukimura O, Gill IS (2009) Image-fusion, augmented reality, and predictive surgical navigation. Urol Clin North Am 36(2):115–123
38. Tan GY, Goel RK, Kaouk JH, Tewari AK (2009) Technological advances in robotic-assisted laparoscopic surgery. Urol Clin North Am 36(2):237–249
39. Archip N, Clatz O, Whalen S, Kacher D, Fedorov A, Kot A, Chrisochoides N, Jolesz F, Golby A, Black PM, Warfield SK (2007) Non-rigid alignment of pre-operative MRI, fMRI, and DT-MRI with intra-operative MRI for enhanced visualization and navigation in image-guided neurosurgery. Neuroimage 35(2):609–624
40. Konishi K, Hashizume M, Nakamoto M, Kakeji Y, Yoshino I, Taketomi A, Sato Y, Tamura S, Maehara Y (2005) Augmented reality navigation system for endoscopic surgery based on three-dimensional ultrasound and computed tomography: application to 20 clinical cases. Int Congress Ser 1281:537–542
41. Boyer B, Le Marec E, Ait-Ameur A, Hauret L, Dion A, Aterii-Tehau C (2003) Tomodensitométrie: principes, formation de l'image. Encycl Méd Chir (Elsevier, Paris), Radiodiagnostic 37-170(A-10):1–16
42. Vargas M, Nguyen D, Viallon M, Delavelle J (2009) Imagerie du plexus brachial (PB). J Radiol 90(10):1448–1448
43. Ben Salem D, Couvreur G, Soichot P, Giroud M, Krausé D, Ricolfi F (2005) Apport de la sequence T2-STIR dans l'exploration des plexopathies brachiales demyelinisantes chroniques. J Radiol 86(10):1249–1249
44. Viallon M, Vargas MI, Jlassi H, Lovblad KO, Delavelle J (2008) High-resolution and functional magnetic resonance imaging of the brachial plexus using an isotropic 3D T2 STIR (Short Term Inversion Recovery) SPACE sequence and diffusion tensor imaging. Eur Radiol 18(5):1018–1023
45. Tagliafico A, Succio G, Neumaier CE, Baio G, Serafini G, Ghidara M, Calabrese M, Martinoli C (2012) Brachial plexus assessment with three-dimensional isotropic resolution fast spin echo MRI: comparison with conventional MRI at 3.0 T. Br J Radiol 85(1014):e110–6
46. Hostettler A, George D, Rémond Y, Nicolau SA, Soler L, Marescaux J (2010) Bulk modulus and volume variation measurement of the liver and the kidneys in vivo using abdominal kinetics during free breathing. Comput Methods Programs Biomed 100(2):149–157
47. Krucker J, Xu S, Glossop N, Viswanathan A, Borgert J, Schulz H, Wood BJ (2007) Electromagnetic tracking for thermal ablation and biopsy guidance: clinical evaluation of spatial accuracy. J Vasc Interv Radiol 18(9):1141–1150
48. Yamanaka Y, Kamogawa J, Katagi R, Kodama K, Misaki H, Kamada K, Okuda S, Morino T, Ogata T, Yamamoto H (2010) 3-D MRI/CT fusion imaging of the lumbar spine. Skeletal Radiol 39(3):285–288

Skin Flaps

16

Thomas Lauwers, Tom Van Mulken, and Darren Booi

16.1 Introduction

Soon after the introduction of robotic surgery, many surgeons looked for an expansion of the potential applications for this device. The feasibility of performing robot-assisted microsurgery was explored in 1998 [10]. From 2005 onwards, multiple articles have been published in this field covering experimental studies [1, 5–7], microdissection [2–4], and more recently, robot-assisted microanastomosis or sutures [3, 11, 13, 16]. Robot-assisted microsurgery was first utilised in our department in 2006 during breast reconstructive surgery in a patient using a deep inferior epigastric perforator (DIEP) flap [15].

The example used for this chapter is a free groin flap.

16.2 Observation

We used a free groin flap to resolve recurrent problems at the donor site of a previous pedicled radial forearm flap to cover a defect on the dorsal hand (Fig. 16.1). Skin graft closure led to tendon adhesions and unstable covering.

The patient was placed in the supine position, with the right arm on a side table. The size and setup of our operating room did not permit installation of the robot whilst operating on both sides of the patient. The robot software was started whilst resecting the skin graft and simultaneous prelevation of the flap starting on the donor site at the left groin whilst preparing the recipient site at the right forearm. After prelevation of the groin flap and debridement of the right forearm, the operating table was turned 90° and the robot installed (Fig. 16.2).

T. Lauwers, M.D. (✉) • T. Van Mulken, M.D. • D. Booi, M.D.
Department of Plastic, Reconstructive and Hand Surgery, University Hospital Maastricht,
P Debyelaan 25, P.O. Box 5800, Maastricht 6202AZ, The Netherlands
e-mail: t.lauwers@mumc.nl

P. Liverneaux et al. (eds.), *Telemicrosurgery*,
DOI 10.1007/978-2-8178-0391-3_16, © Springer-Verlag France 2013

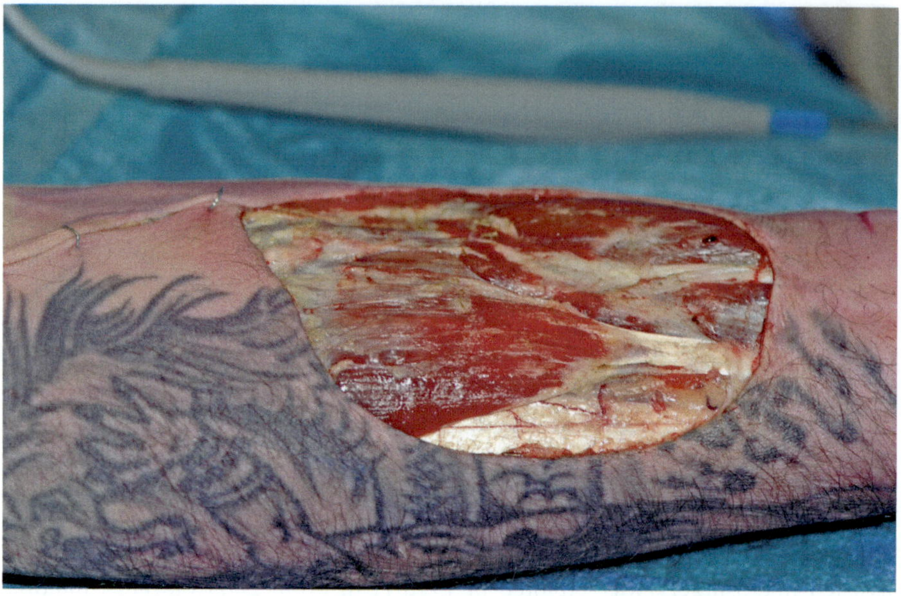

Fig. 16.1 Defect in the right forearm after resection of the unstable covering

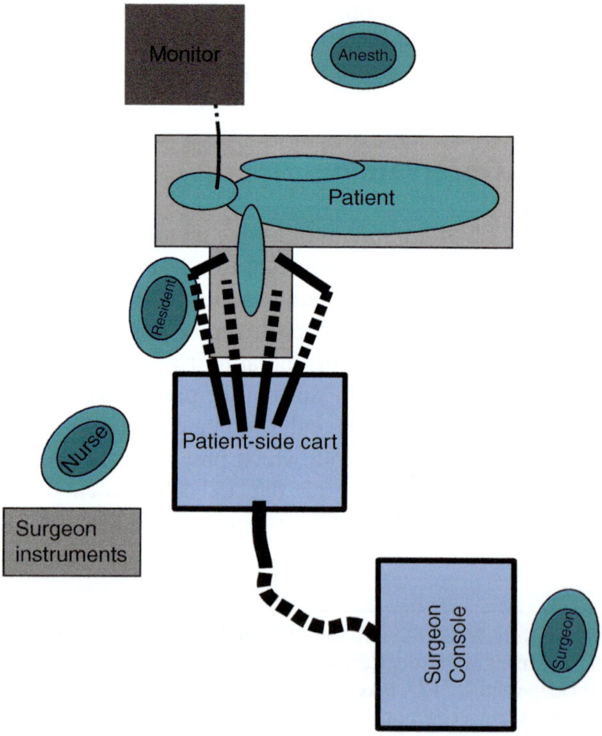

Fig. 16.2 Da Vinci SI® robot (Intuitive Surgical™, Sunnyvale, CA, USA) on the caudal side of the arm table and assistant and nurse on the cranial side of the arm table

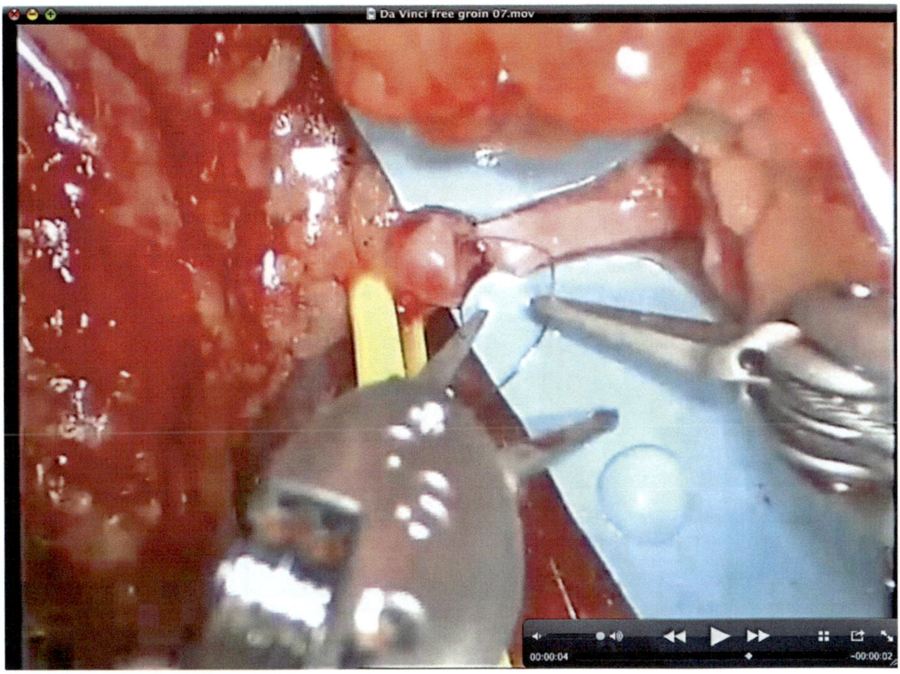

Fig. 16.3 Vidcap of the microsurgical suture, a stitch

The size of the donor vessels were an arterial diameter of 2.0 mm and a vein of equal size anastomosed to the stump of the radial artery previously transected and now further freed by robot-assisted surgery. Set-up time and sterile draping of the robot was 10 min, whilst the flap remained on its pedicle as control. A 30° optics, three arms with two Black Diamond® forceps, and one Potts scissors were used. Setting for motion, scaling was set to "Extra Fine" being 5:1. Anastomoses were carried out with polypropylene monofilament 9/0 (Prolene®) (Fig. 16.3). Ischaemia lasted 45 min, mainly due to difficult arterial anastomosis on a radialis stump that was transected 2 years before. There was a clear but not excessive mismatch in diameter of both the arterial and venous anastomoses of about 1.0 mm (Fig. 16.4). This was resolved with two mattress sutures (Fig. 16.5).

16.3 Discussion

Whilst performing microsurgery and microanastomoses with a robot, several specific aspects have to be taken into account. Most important are the quality of the three-dimensional (3D) image and the lack of haptic feedback. To a lesser extent, the practical aspects of working with a 5:1, downscaling of movements and particularities of the robotic instruments are also important and are discussed.

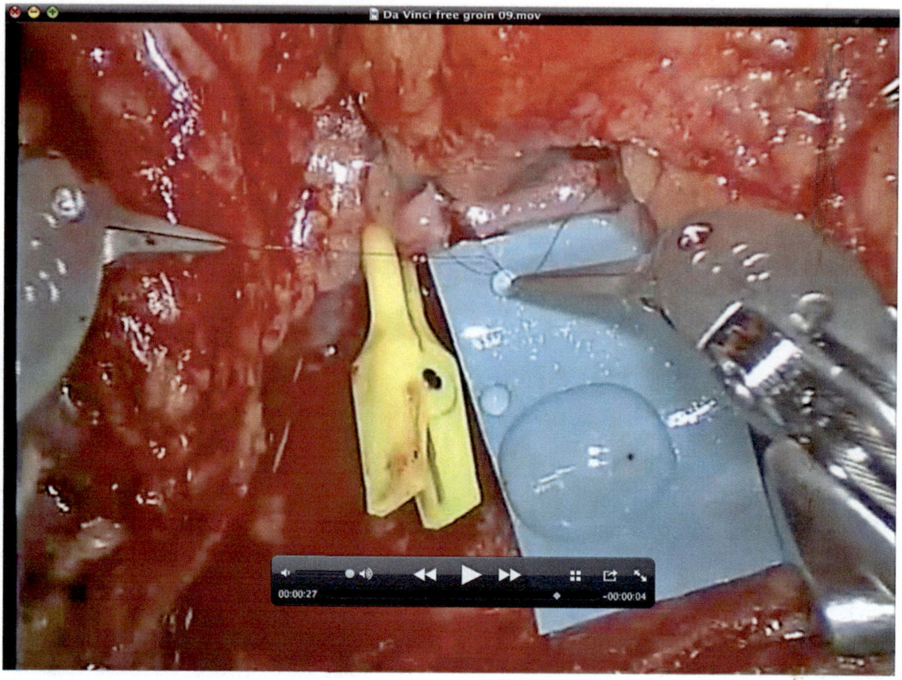

Fig. 16.4 Vidcap of the microsurgical suture, a knot

First is the relative quality of 3D vision. Although it certainly has better in-depth view, it is not as accurate as a normal view. Three-dimensional vision is comparable to a classic surgical microscope and is better than an endoscope but still not the "real thing." Just as is the case for endoscopy or surgery using a microscope, there is a learning curve for the handling of instruments. This means that in very demanding conditions like prelevation of a flap or making a microanastomosis, one has to move with great caution, even with a motion scaling setting of 5:1. The probing of instruments in the deep end of the wound can potentially cause damage.

Second is the absence of haptic feedback. The relative importance of lack of haptic feedback is a controversial issue [8, 9, 12]. Many articles have been published stressing both the importance of haptic feedback and proposing models to solve the problem. On the contrary, many other published articles have stated that visual feedback is sufficient. This debate is ongoing [14]. The absence of haptic feedback is not a major problem in performing microvascular anastomosis. Visual feedback is sufficient to handle the tissue and prevent intimal damage and undue tension. It is notable that articles stating the need of haptic feedback used tests with suture of relative important thickness (e.g. 6/0), whilst experience shows that with decreasing suture calibre, the estimated point of breaking feeling gets less accurate. The absence of haptic feedback is not so much a problem for suture handling but could pose a problem in the manipulation of needles used for microsurgery. Tissue manipulation is not dependent on haptic feedback. Even in traditional microsurgery,

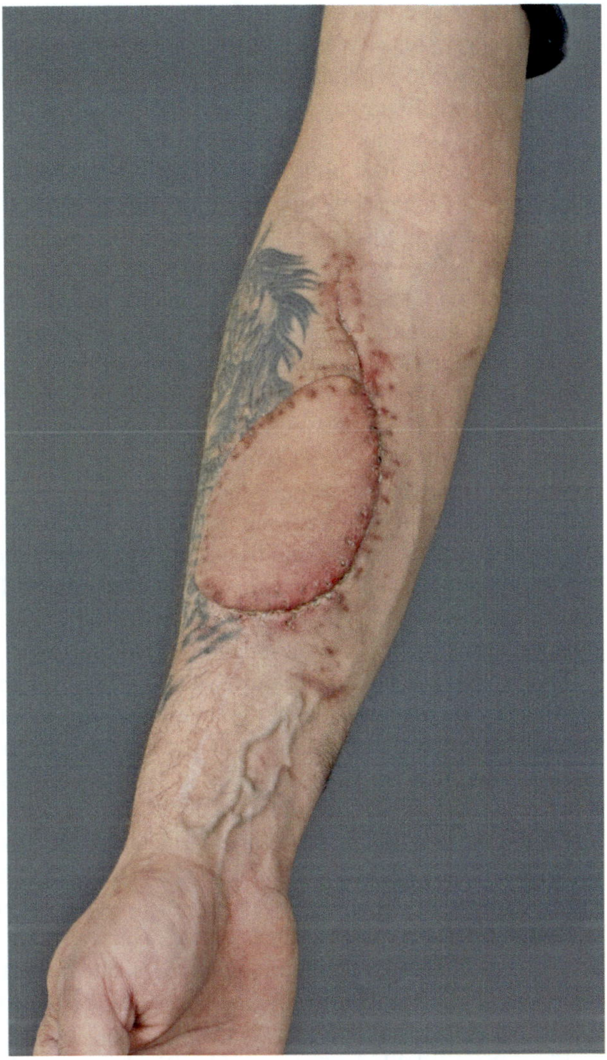

Fig. 16.5 Result after 6 weeks

haptic feedback is not the main method one relies on to decide whether too much traction exists during suturing; by the time one feels tissues of that size or thickness rupturing, the damage is usually already done. One is therefore trained to see the stretching of the tissue and loosen tension before rupture occurs. The handling of sutures and needles is more problematic. Whilst passing the wire from one clamp to the other in order to have the needle in the clamp, the brief moment of tension that results could lead to breaking of the suture. The grasping and positioning of a needle in a Black Diamond® forceps is most often possible by using soft tissue as a rotation point, exactly the way we do when positioning our needle when we cannot let go of the instrument in the other hand. Sometimes this does not lead to a satisfactory position of the needle necessitating the use of both clamps to place the needle in the needle holder. This carries a risk of bending or even breaking of the needle if repositioning is made without releasing of one or both clamps. It is not impossible though, and we do it relatively frequently but with a lot of attention to the timing of grasping, releasing and pushing the right position.

The combination of both disadvantages described above has the following consequences: (1) It can sometimes lead to unwanted traction or pushing on the needle or even the anastomosis when both instruments are crossed one over the other in the centre of the visual field. Whilst one does not see the underlying instrument, it could push or pull on the anastomosis or the needle or suture wire. Hence, crossing of the instruments without constant visual control of the vital structures is to be avoided. (2) The freedom of movement of the arms of the robot is greater than that of the camera in zooming in or out. There is therefore a possibility of placing instruments out of the field of vision. Whilst this can be merely challenging for organising an operating field, it can also be dangerous as there is also a lack of haptic feedback (in contrast to laparoscopic surgery for instance).

In conclusion, haptic feedback in itself is not necessary to perform microsurgery but may be essential to prevent tissue damage around the operation field or in depth whilst operating in a deep or endoscopic environment. This is a typical problem for microsurgery where the field of vision is very narrow as maximal zoom is necessarily applied to obtain maximal magnification.

Downscaling means larger movements at the surgeon console than in the operating field by the patient-side cart. When larger movements have to be performed at the operating field, this could result in "fighting" of the master controls and their articulations. If there is discrepancy in the visual feedback (e.g. zooming in and moving at the edge of the field of vision), one cannot always differentiate between a block at the console or at the patient-side cart as it is not immediately obvious that the blocking occurs at the console and not between instruments in the operating field. A simple clutch and repositioning solves the problem. It is simply part of the learning curve to have this reflex.

Two aspects of instrumentation do complicate the use of a surgical robot to assist microsurgery and to a higher degree microsurgical suturing: (1) the available instruments and their behaviour and (2) the price tag.

First, the available instruments like Black Diamond® forceps and Pott scissors® as available for the da Vinci® system (Intuitive Surgical™, Sunnyvale, CA, USA) are suitable for microsurgery but have their limitations concerning the diameter of structures that can be manipulated safely. Furthermore, the range of instruments is very limited, and many instruments that are widely used in traditional microsurgery do not yet exist in the repertorium of robot-assisted microsurgery instruments. Most evident examples are dilators, surgical non-traumatising forceps, different scissors (such as angled or nerve scissors), arteriotomy clamps and vascular clip clamps. This lack of choice is mainly due to the fact that these instruments have not yet been developed. Another point of interest whilst performing microanastomoses is the "locking" of Black Diamond forceps in a clenched position. This is experienced by several users of the system, although the reasons for this remain unclear. This can result in dangerous consequences whilst dilating vessels as opening of the forceps might be sudden and complete. Hence, the development of a dilator is mandatory, although not sufficient for the safe dilatation of vessels. Until that time, the back of two needles can be used to dilate. The relevance of ongoing research and development of more suitable instruments for existing robots, might be lessened by the development of dedicated robots, possessing their own microsurgery instruments or manipulating existing instruments for manual microsurgery.

The cost plays a role as well. Every instrument can only be used ten times before mandatory replacement. The use of multiple instruments in the course of one intervention could become very expensive. Nevertheless, finer and more divers instruments will be essential for the further development of robot-assisted microsurgery.

Conclusion

Presently, microsurgery can be done and microanastomoses successfully performed to a given diameter of vessels. This is not a mere novelty but can be expected to evolve into a surgical tool adding to our problem solving capacities.

The installation of the robotic system is certainly time-consuming and requires more routine care and specialisation from the nursing staff than does a conventional operating microscope. One could imagine in the future patients being operated from a distance by highly skilled specialists, with a nurse and assistant surgeon present at a remote patient location. This could provide more specialised care to a larger region. Installing the robot will always be quicker, easier, less risky, and cheaper than transferring the patient.

Second, in the future, great benefit can be derived from the further development of endoscopic microsurgery, to a certain degree already available for gynaecology, cardiac surgery, and laryngeal surgery but more than probably of interest to plexus surgery or other more deeply localised anastomosis, which could in fact ease the selection of suitable vessels and minimise surgical trauma. Free flap reconstruction for defects in the thorax and perineal region could benefit from deeply placed microanastomosis as this makes further dissection to reach vessels unnecessary.

The evolution of robot-assisted microsurgery (telemicrosurgery) and the training will surely resemble that of laparoscopic surgery 20 years ago. There has been a lot of distrust and some enthusiasm in the beginning, but very soon residents who are trained from the beginning of their careers might outclass their mentors. There are indications that residents and trainees will pick up this technique quickly [5].

References

1. Bourges JL, Hubschman JP, Burt B et al (2009) Robotic microsurgery: corneal transplantation. Br J Ophthalmol 93:1672–1675
2. Boyd B, Umansky J, Samson M et al (2006) Robotic harvest of internal mammary vessels in breast reconstruction. J Reconstr Microsurg 22:261–266

3. Caillet M, Vandromme J, Rozenberg S et al (2010) Robotically assisted laparoscopic microsurgical tubal reanastomosis: a retrospective study. Fertil Steril 94:1844–1847
4. Csókay A, Valálik I, Jobbágy A (2009) Early experiences with a novel (robot hand) technique in the course of microneurosurgery. Surg Neurol 71:469–472
5. Karamanoukian RL, Bui T, McConnell MP et al (2006) Transfer of training in robotic-assisted microvascular surgery. Ann Plast Surg 57:662–665
6. Katz R, Taylor J, Rosson G et al (2006) Robotics in plastic and reconstructive surgery: use of a telemanipulator slave robot to perform microvascular anastomoses. J Reconstr Microsurg 22:53–57
7. Katz RD, Rosson GD, Taylor JA et al (2005) Robotics in microsurgery: use of a surgical robot to perform a free flap in a pig. Microsurgery 25:566–569
8. King CH, Culjat MO, Franco ML et al (2009) A multi-element tactile feedback system for robot-assisted minimally invasive surgery. IEEE Trans Haptics 2:52–56
9. King CH, Culjat MO, Franco ML et al (2009) Tactile feedback induces reduced grasping force in robotic surgery. IEEE Trans Haptics 2:103–110
10. Margossian H, Garcia-Ruiz A, Falcone T et al (1998) Robotically assisted laparoscopic microsurgical uterine horn anastomosis. Fertil Steril 70:530–534
11. Nectoux E, Taleb C, Liverneaux P (2009) Nerve repair in telemicrosurgery: an experimental study. J Reconstr Microsurg 25:261–265
12. Panchulidze I, Berner S, Mantovani G et al (2011) Is haptic feedback necessary to microsurgical suturing? Comparative study of 9/0 and 10/0 knot tying operated by 24 surgeons. Hand Surg 16:1–3
13. Parekattil SJ, Atalah HN, Cohen MS (2010) Video technique for human robot-assisted microsurgical vasovasostomy. J Endourol 24:511–514
14. Sangpradit K, Liu H, Dasgupta P et al (2011) Finite element modelling of soft tissue rolling indentation. IEEE Trans Biomed Eng 58:3319–3327
15. Van der Hulst RR, Sawor J, Bouvy NJ (2007) Microvascular anastomosis: is there a role for robotic sugery? J Plast Reconstr Aesthet Surg 60:101–102
16. Woo YJ (2006) Robotic cardiac surgery. Int J Med Robotics Comput Assist Surg 2:225–232

Muscle Flaps

17

Jesse Creed Selber and John C. Pedersen

17.1 Introduction

Free and pedicled muscle flaps have been in use by plastic surgeons for a variety of applications since World War I and remain workhorses in scalp, extremity, head and neck, and breast reconstruction. Harvest of muscle flaps traditionally requires incisions that allow access to muscle origin, insertion, and pedicle. Because some muscles such as the latissimus dorsi and rectus abdominis are large, incisions can be anywhere from 20 to 30 cm in length. These donor sites are conspicuously located on the abdomen and back and are the source of morbidity in the form of cosmesis, seroma, and hernia. Because of the desirability of minimally invasive harvest, endoscopic and laparoscopic techniques have been attempted but have not achieved broad acceptance due to technical challenges related to exposure, retraction, and lack of appropriately precise instrumentation.

The robotic interface has supplied the necessary exposure and picture clarity through high resolution, three-dimensional optics, and the necessary precision instrumentation through wristed motion at the instrument tips to accomplish both muscle and pedicle dissection. For this reason, robotic muscle harvest, although still in its infancy, holds excellent promise in reducing donor site morbidity for these common reconstructive procedures.

J.C. Selber, M.D., M.P.H. (✉)
Department of Plastic Surgery – Unit 1488, Anderson Cancer Center,
The University of Texas, M.D., 1400 Pressler St., Houston 77030, TX, USA
e-mail: jcselber@mdanderson.org

J.C. Pedersen, M.D., F.A.C.S.
Department of Plastic Surgery,
Akron Plastic Surgeons, Akron, OH, USA
e-mail: solstadwest@me.com

P. Liverneaux et al. (eds.), *Telemicrosurgery*,
DOI 10.1007/978-2-8178-0391-3_17, © Springer-Verlag France 2013

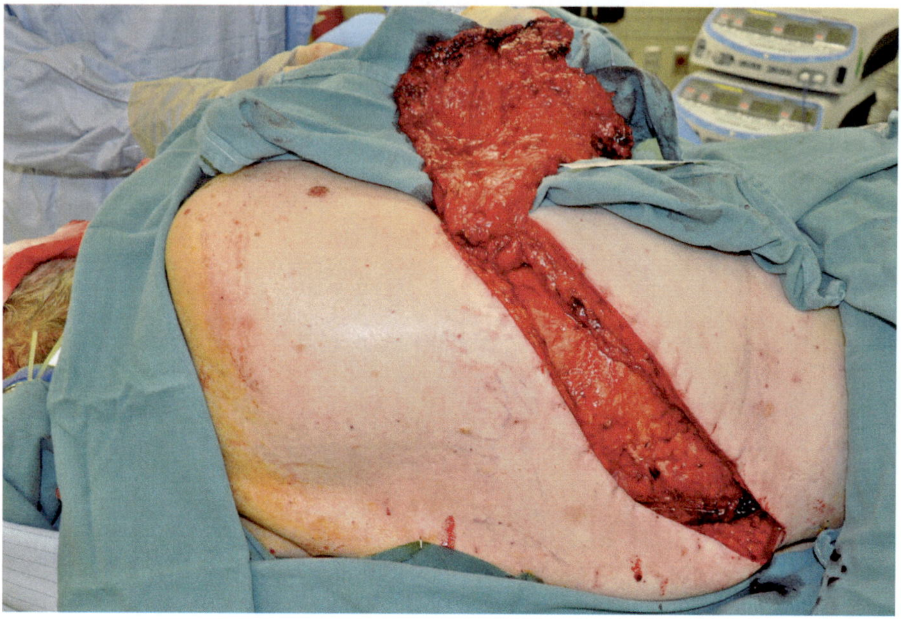

Fig. 17.1 The latissimus dorsi muscle has been a workhorse of reconstructive surgery since its original description by Iginio Tansini in 1897. Traditional harvest technique involves an incision on the back measuring between 15 and 25 cm. An example is shown here. This donor site scar is typically unsightly and represents the primary objection to undergoing this operation and primary area of dissatisfaction following it

17.2 Latissimus Dorsi

The latissimus dorsi muscle has been a workhorse of reconstructive surgery since its original description by Iginio Tansini in 1897 [23]. Its diverse applications range from breast salvage, immediate breast reconstruction with implant, partial breast reconstruction, chest wall and intrathoracic reconstruction, scalp and extremity coverage, and functional muscle transfer [2, 4, 8, 13, 14, 20, 21]. Traditional harvest technique involves an incision on the back measuring between 15 and 25 cm (Fig. 17.1). This donor site scar is typically unsightly and represents the primary objection to undergoing this operation and primary area of dissatisfaction following it.

Minimally invasive harvest of the latissimus has long been a desirable goal. Endoscopic harvest has been attempted by multiple groups and is still practiced in certain centers [12, 15, 16]. But because of technical challenges such as line of sight around the curvature of the back, limitations of endoscopic instrumentation, and difficulty maintaining an optical window, all but a few centers have abandoned this technique [7, 17].

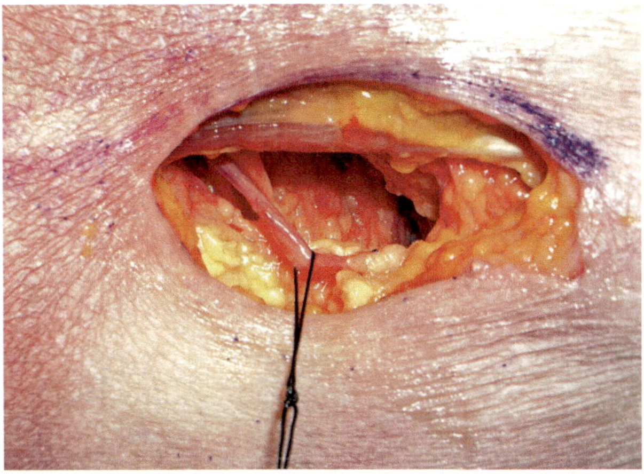

Fig. 17.2 An initial 5-cm axillary incision is made beginning at the axillary crease, along the posterior axillary fold. From this incision, the thoracodorsal pedicle is identified and dissected. A vessel loop is placed around it for ease of visualization during later robotic dissection. Using electrocautery and a lighted retractor, the anterior border of the latissimus muscle is dissected free along most of its length

17.2.1 Operative Procedure

The patient is placed in the decubitus position, with hips at the break in the bed. The foot is then dropped to open up the torso between the rib cage and the pelvis. An initial 5-cm axillary incision is made beginning at the axillary crease, along the posterior axillary fold. From this incision, the thoracodorsal pedicle is identified and dissected (Fig. 17.2). A vessel loop is placed around it for ease of visualization during later robotic dissection. Using electrocautery and a lighted retractor, the anterior border of the latissimus muscle is dissected free along most of its length. An area approximately 5 cm anterior to the border of the muscle is also dissected in order to create a potential space for robotic port placement. Next, a balloon dilator (AutoSuture Spacemaker Plus®, Covidien™, Mansfield, MA, USA) is placed under the muscle, distal to the pedicle and along the long axis of the muscle, and inflated to assist in submuscular dissection (Fig. 17.3). The axillary incision is then temporarily closed over a 12-mm port with a running locking suture, to maintain insufflation.

Markings for the ports are made, starting about 15 cm from the axillary fold. The first port introduced is the 12-mm camera port. A 1-cm incision is made approximately 23 cm from the axillary fold and 6–7 cm anterior to the anterior border of the muscle. The port is placed under direct vision through the axillary incision. The proximal, 5-mm port is then placed under direct vision approximately four finger breadths (8 cm) proximal to the camera port (Fig. 17.4). The zero degree endoscope is introduced and the distal, 5-mm port is placed approximately four finger breadths distal to the camera port and slightly anterior to it, under endoscopic vision (Fig. 17.5).

Following port placement, the robotic side cart is positioned on the back side of the bed and the arms are brought over the patient and into position, nearly parallel to the plane of the floor (Fig. 17.6). The ports are docked, and insufflation is applied at 8–10 mmHg. Dissection begins along the under surface of the muscle. If dissection

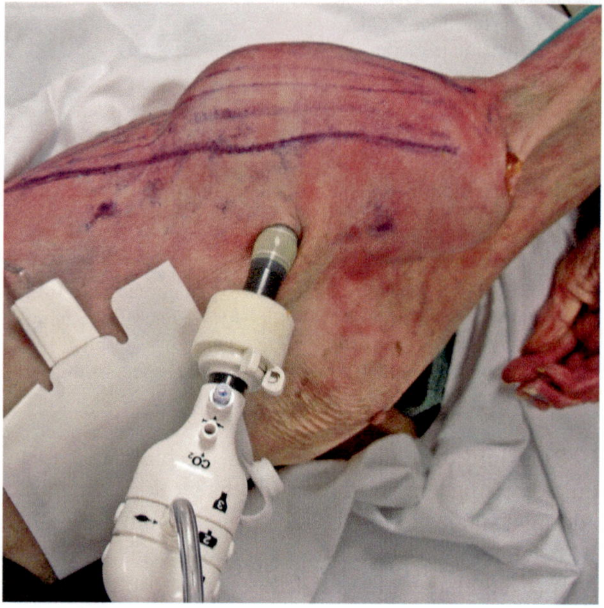

Fig. 17.3 A balloon dilator (AutoSuture Spacemaker Plus®, Covidien™, Mansfield, MA, USA) is placed under the muscle, distal to the pedicle and along the long axis of the muscle, and inflated to assist in submuscular dissection

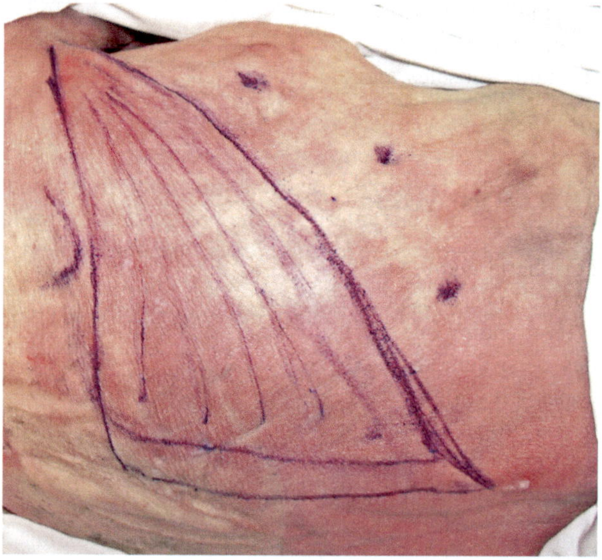

Fig. 17.4 The ports are located at approximately 15, 23, and 31 cm from the axillary fold, and approximately 5, 6, and 5 cm from the anterior border of the latissimus muscle, respectively

began along the subcutaneous plane, it would be impossible to maintain the optical window beneath the muscle because insufflation would press the muscle down against the chest wall. Monopolar scissors and Codier® grasper (Intuitive Surgical™, Sunnyvale, CA, USA) are used for the dissection. After the undersurface of the muscle is dissected to the borders, the grasper is used to pull the anterior edge of the muscle down, and dissection proceeds over the superficial surface of the muscle.

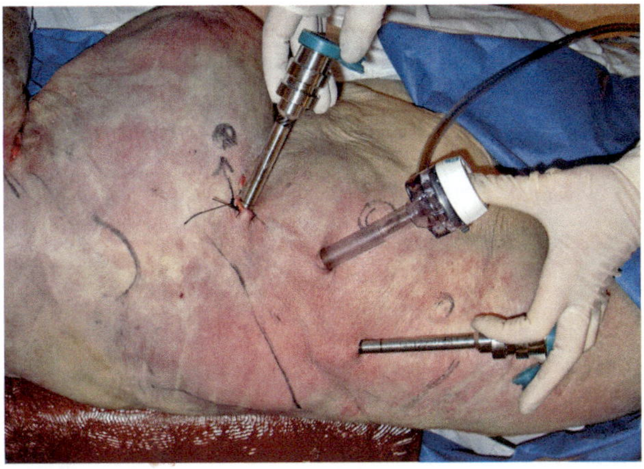

Fig. 17.5 The first port introduced is the 12-mm camera port. The port is placed under direct vision through the axillary incision. The proximal, 5-mm port is then placed under direct vision approximately four finger breadths (8 cm) proximal to the camera port. The zero-degree endoscope is introduced and the distal, 5-mm port is placed approximately four finger breadths distal to the camera port and slightly anterior to it, under endoscopic vision

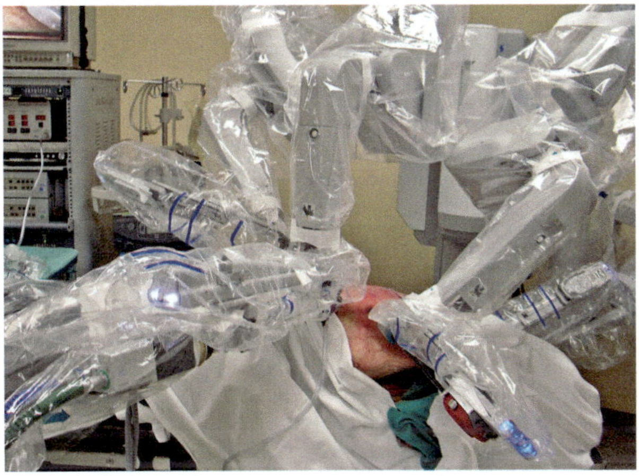

Fig. 17.6 Following port placement, the robotic side cart is positioned on the back side of the bed and the arms are brought over the patient and into position, nearly parallel to the plane of the floor

Once dissection is complete along both the deep and superficial surface, the monopolar scissors is used to take the muscle off the inferior-posterior border (Fig. 17.7). If it is a right muscle, the scissors is placed in the arm corresponding to the left hand. If it is the left muscle, the monopolar scissors is reversed. This allows the surgeon to dissect from inferior to superior. As the muscle is released, it is pushed up toward the axilla in order to maintain the tension and visualization along the posterior border. Once the muscle has been liberated proximal to the tip of the scapula, the muscle will be easily accessible through the axillary incision. This incision is then opened, and the muscle is delivered (Fig. 17.8). The robot is undocked, drains are placed in the port sites, and the axillary incision is closed.

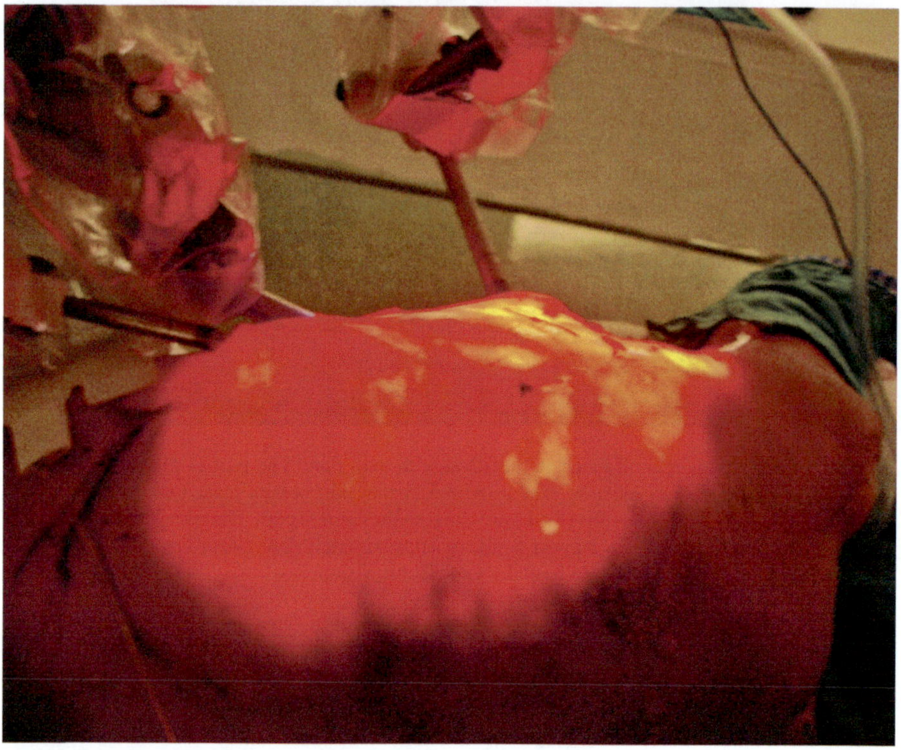

Fig. 17.7 Insufflation and transillumination show the area of subcutaneous dissection for the latissimus dorsi muscle

17.2.2 Technical Considerations

There are several technical considerations that facilitate a successful dissection. A smooth and effortless dissection relies completely on an optimized setup. If the setup has been well conceived, the dissection is easily executed. If the setup is poorly planned, the dissection is a struggle.

1. For positioning, the patient's hips should be at the break in the bed, and the head and foot should be dropped several inches. The reason for this is the most distal arm has to drop down almost parallel to the patient in order to achieve the appropriate angle for submuscular dissection and release of the muscle inferiorly. If the bed is flat, this arm will collide with the prominence of the hip and make dissection difficult.
2. During the initial axillary dissection, as much of the anterior border of the muscle should be dissected as possible. This greatly facilitates subsequent robotic dissection, which proceeds from anterior to posterior and relies on easy identification of the muscle within the fat. Also, the portion of the anterior border of muscle closest to the camera port is awkward to release because of its proximity to the camera itself; thus, open dissection of this lip of muscle facilitates this awkward part of the dissection.

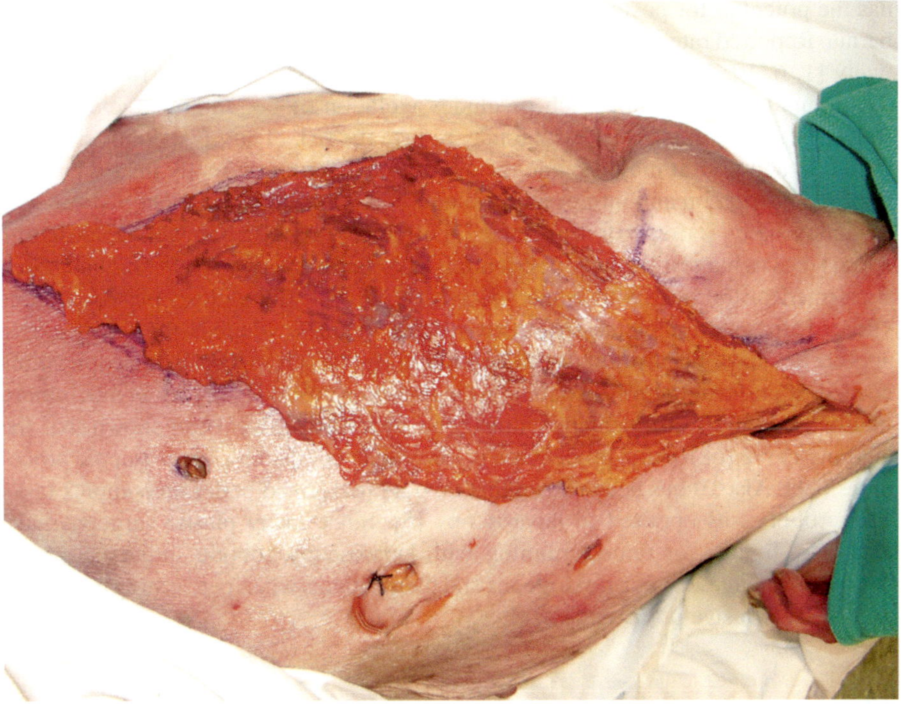

Fig. 17.8 Once the muscle has been liberated proximal to the tip of the scapula, the muscle will be easily accessible through the axillary incision. This incision is then opened, and the muscle is delivered

3. Adequate space must be made anterior to the muscle so that the ports are far enough away to avoid collisions among the instruments and arms as they angle toward the proximal and distal extremes of the dissection.
4. The space for the ports should be confluent: any soft tissue connections between the ports will obscure the optical window.
5. When dissection over the muscle reaches the midpoint between the posterior axillary line and the spine, the curve of the rib cage is at its greatest. At this point, it is often useful to switch to a 30° down scope in order to complete the posterior dissection.

If these suggestions are followed, robotic dissection of the latissimus is a reliable and reproducible technique. Incisions are minimized, and drains can be brought out the port sites so these stab incisions are not wasted.

17.3 Rectus Abdominis

Access to the rectus abdominis muscle has traditionally been via a long, vertical paramedian skin incision, followed by vertical division of the anterior rectus sheath along the length of the entire muscle. This approach is cosmetically undesirable and has the potential for postoperative wound infection, seroma, abdominal bulge, and hernia. Reported rates of bulge and hernia rates are 1.7–4 % and 0.85–2.9 %, respectively [1, 6, 10, 22]. Surgical site morbidity may be as high as 8.5–14.3 % [1, 6]. A minimally invasive approach precludes violation of the anterior rectus sheath from costal margin to pubis, which may reduce the risk of surgical donor site morbidity. In addition, it may provide the ability to perform minimally invasive pelvic floor reconstruction and intraperitoneal, microvascular reconstruction.

Endoscopic extraperitoneal and traditional transperitoneal laparoscopic approaches to harvest the rectus abdominis muscle for free tissue transfer have been performed in the past with some success [3, 9, 18]. The endoscopic procedures violated the anterior rectus sheath to varying degrees, whereas the laparoscopic approaches have been primarily been limited by the advanced laparoscopic skills needed to perform them. In contrast to laparoscopy, robotic surgery is much more intuitive and the instrumentation much less awkward. It has been shown that the learning curve for robotic procedures is lower than comparable laparoscopic procedures [11]. Also, it has been shown that novices performed better on complex tasks using robotics as opposed to laparoscopy [5]. Since many plastic surgeons have either no, limited, or remote training with laparoscopy, robotic surgery has even clearer advantages for plastic surgeons and their patients when performing advanced, minimally invasive procedures.

17.3.1 Operative Technique

All ports are placed contralateral to the side of the muscle being harvested. The first port is placed approximately 7 cm lateral to the rectus abdominis, in line with the umbilicus with a Hassan cannula technique. Carbon dioxide insufflation is initiated and pneumoperitoneum maintained at 15 mmHg. A 30° Vision System scope is then placed, and under endoscopic vision, the second and third ports are placed. The second port is positioned 4 cm inferior to the costal margin and 5 cm lateral to semilunar line. The third port is placed 4 cm superior to the anterior superior iliac spine and 5 cm lateral to the semilunar line (Fig. 17.9). Port 1 is used exclusively for the Vision System, which consists of a 30° up angled three-dimensional scope. Ports 2 and 3 are used for dissection and retraction. Instrumentation includes the monopolar spatula and PK dissecting forceps. Instruments in ports 2 and 3 are interchanged as needed throughout the case.

The approach is initiated by incising the posterior rectus sheath and peritoneum immediately lateral to the linea alba, just off the midline. The avascular plane posterior to the rectus abdominis is dissected, separating the muscle from the fascia. Minimal cautery is used during this part of the dissection. The lateral edge of the rectus abdominis and the intercostal perforators are easily identified and ligated with the PK dissector. After posterior and lateral dissection are completed along the length of the muscle, the dissection between the anterior rectus sheath and rectus abdominis muscle is initiated at the level of the umbilicus. The free muscle planes between inscriptions are predominantly avascular and dissection is accomplished

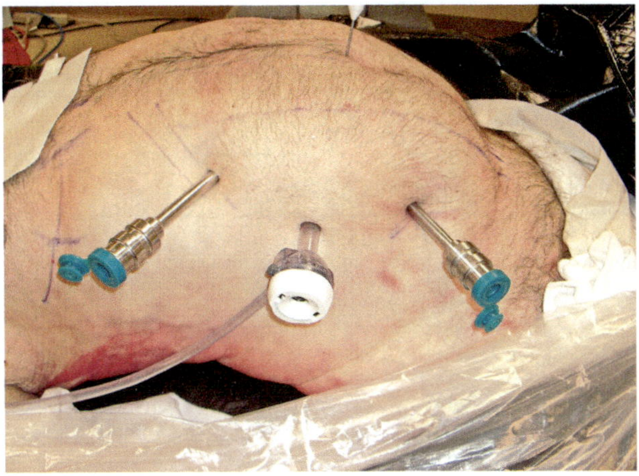

Fig. 17.9 All ports are placed contralateral to the side of the muscle being harvested. The first port is placed approximately 7 cm lateral to the rectus abdominis, in line with the umbilicus with a Hassan cannula technique. Carbon dioxide insufflation is initiated and pneumoperitoneum maintained at 15 mmHg. A 30° Vision System scope is then placed, and under endoscopic vision, the second and third ports are placed. The second port is positioned 4 cm inferior to the costal margin and 5 cm lateral to semilunar line. The third port is placed 4 cm superior to the anterior superior iliac spine and 5 cm lateral to the semilunar line

bluntly with minimal monopolar cautery. Perforating vessels from the deep inferior epigastric artery are easily seen as the muscle hangs between inscriptions. Vessels are ligated using the PK dissector. After both sides of an inscription are dissected free, the camera is brought in for a high magnification view and the monopolar blade is used to dissect the muscle free at the inscriptions. The cephalad-most aspect of the rectus abdominis muscle is divided with monopolar cautery and PK dissector. The division of the rectus abdominis muscle from the pubic symphysis is performed with monopolar cautery, as the tendinous attachment is relatively avascular. The pedicle is then gently dissected down to the external iliac artery.

The anterior abdominal wall is transilluminated using the light source on the Vision System to help place the skin incision used to harvest the freed rectus muscle. A 2.5-cm incision is made in the anterior rectus sheath to externalize the muscle (Fig. 17.10). The anterior rectus sheath is closed with interrupted 0-Prolene sutures. The posterior rectus sheath and peritoneum are left open.

17.4 Case Report

Thirty-year-old female presented for right lower extremity limb salvage. Her medical history is remarkable for reticular cell sarcoma of the right lower thigh that was treated with resection and followed by chemotherapy and radiation therapy. The lower leg musculature as a result had become atrophic but remained highly functional as the patient was able to run and had completed a marathon. To maintain her

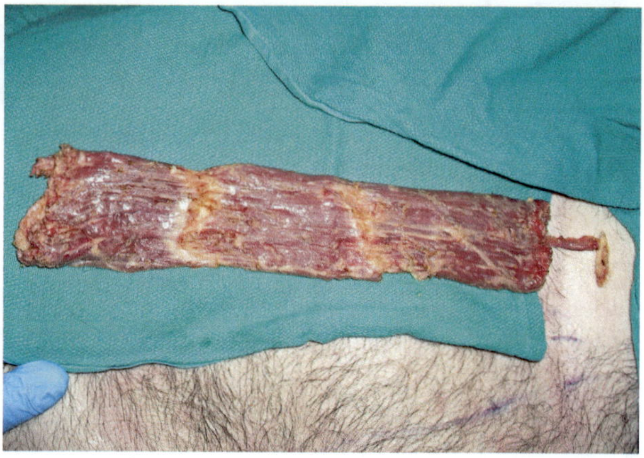

Fig. 17.10 The anterior abdominal wall is transilluminated using the light source on the Vision System to help place the skin incision used to harvest the freed rectus muscle. A 2.5-cm incision is made in the anterior rectus sheath to externalize the muscle

active lifestyle, she underwent several procedures for limb lengthening, and most recently due to worsening arthritis, she underwent a right knee arthroplasty out of state. Two months after her knee surgery, the skin incision dehisced, and she developed hardware-related infection. Subsequently, she underwent washout and debridement of the right knee with polyethylene insert exchange and V.A.C.® placement (KCI™, San Antonio, TX, USA). There was no local muscle available as her native leg musculature was atrophied, so the decision was made to use rectus abdominis muscle free flap and the distal superficial femoral artery as conduit for limb salvage. After the muscle was harvested as described above, it was anastomosed to the distal superficial femoral artery in an end to side fashion using a surgical microscope and standard microvascular technique, providing well-vascularized tissue over the exposed tendon and bone. Her port placement, closed incisions, and postoperative donor sites are shown (Figs. 17.11, 17.12, and 17.13).

Conclusion

The precision and enhanced imaging technology of robotic surgery has allowed minimally invasive procedures to be extended to surgical procedures that may be too technically complex for laparoscopic or endoscopic techniques. The robotic approaches that we describe, although not in widespread clinical use, are relatively straightforward and reproducible techniques for accomplishing muscle harvest without significant donor site morbidity. Both approaches take advantage of insufflation, gravity, precision instrumentation, and three-dimensional imaging with multiple angle scopes.

Just as there are advantages, there are disadvantages. The intraperitoneal approach to the rectus abdominis adds all of the risks and potential complications related to accessing and working in the peritoneal cavity, such as bowel injury, adhesion formation, and hernia. The latissimus dorsi approach increases the theoretical risk of pneumothorax and pedicle damage if inadvertently encountered.

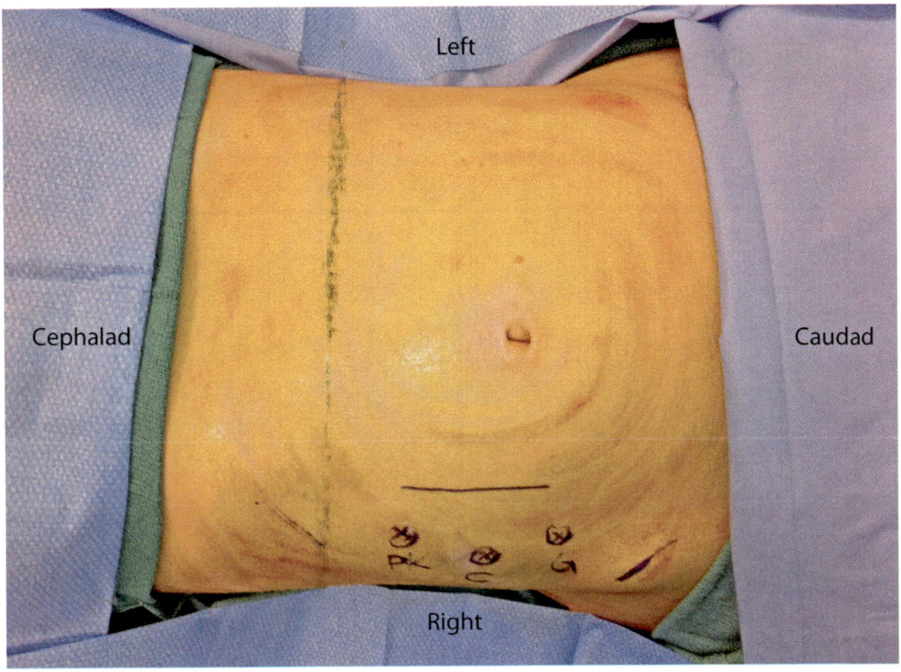

Fig. 17.11 30-year-old female presented for right lower extremity limb salvage. A robotic rectus was planned. The port sites were marked preoperatively

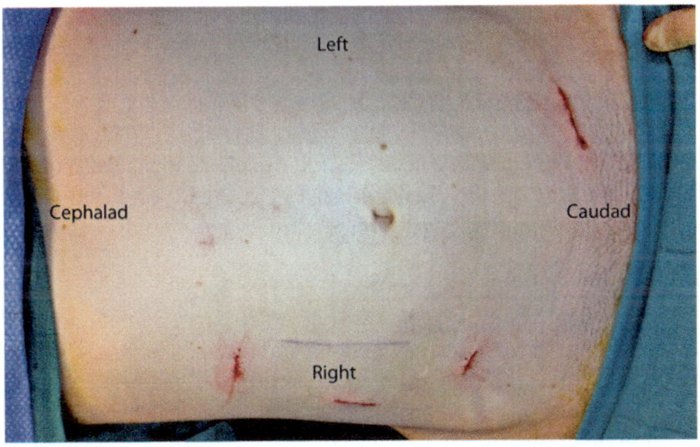

Fig. 17.12 After robotic harvest, port sites were closed. The immediate postoperative appearance is shown

Also, the robotic approach is more costly, although this effect may be obviated by decreased surgical site morbidity and length of stay [19].

Overall, robotic muscle harvest represents a tremendous step forward in the ongoing quest to minimize donor site morbidity without compromising outcomes in reconstructive surgery.

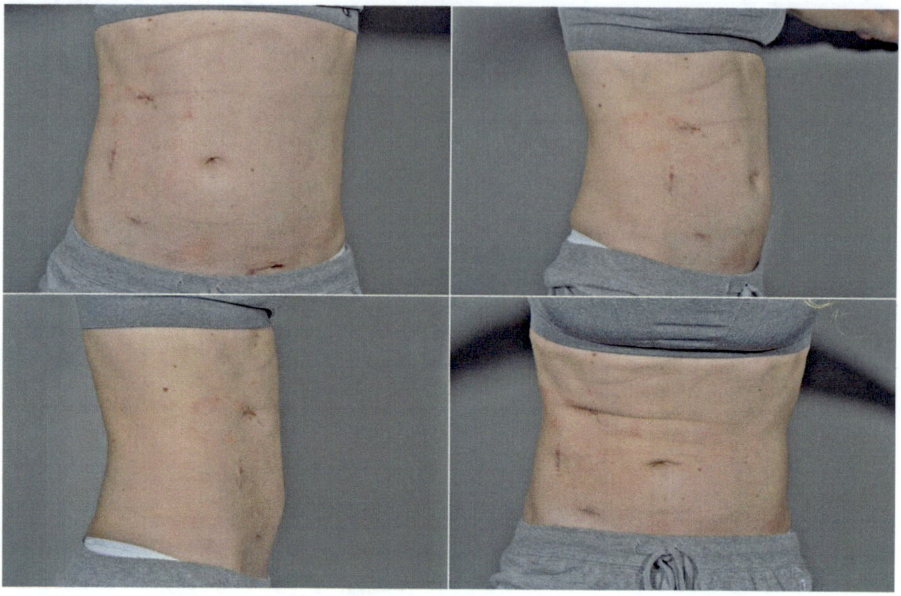

Fig. 17.13 At 1 month postoperatively, her port sites are well healed, and she has no appreciable abdominal dysfunction

References

1. Ascherman JA, Seruya M, Bartsich SA (2008) Abdominal wall morbidity following unilateral and bilateral breast reconstruction with pedicled TRAM flaps: an outcomes analysis of 117 consecutive patients. Plast Reconstr Surg 121:1–8
2. Bartlett SP, May JW Jr, Yaremchuk MJ (1981) The latissimus dorsi muscle: a fresh cadaver study of the primary neurovascular pedicle. Plast Reconstr Surg 67:631–636
3. Bass LS, Karp NS, Benacquista T et al (1995) Endoscopic harvest of the rectus abdominis free flap: balloon dissection in the fascial plane. Ann Plast Surg 34:274–279; discussion 279–280
4. Bostwick J 3rd, Vasconez LO, Jurkiewicz MJ (1978) Breast reconstruction after a radical mastectomy. Plast Reconstr Surg 61:682–693
5. Chandra V, Nehra D, Parent R et al (2010) A comparison of laparoscopic and robotic assisted suturing performance by experts and novices. Surgery 147:830–839
6. Chun YS, Sinha I, Turko A et al (2010) Comparison of morbidity, functional outcome, and satisfaction following bilateral TRAM versus bilateral DIEP flap breast reconstruction. Plast Reconstr Surg 126:1133–1141
7. Fine NA, Orgill DP, Pribaz JJ (1994) Early clinical experience in endoscopic-assisted muscle flap harvest. Ann Plast Surg 33:465–469; discussion 469–472
8. Germann G, Waag KL, Selle B et al (2006) Extremity salvage with a free musculocutaneous latissimus dorsi flap and free tendon transfer after resection of a large congenital fibro sarcoma in a 15-week-old infant. A case report. Microsurgery 26:429–431
9. Greensmith A, Januszkiewicz J, Poole G (2000) Rectus abdominis muscle free flap harvest by laparoscopic sheath-sparing technique. Plast Reconstr Surg 105:1438–1441
10. Kroll SS, Schusterman MA, Reece GP et al (1995) Abdominal wall strength, bulging, and hernia after TRAM flap breast reconstruction. Plast Reconstr Surg 96:616–619

11. Lim PC, Kang E, Park DH (2010) A comparative detail analysis of the learning curve and surgical outcome for robotic hysterectomy with lymphadenectomy versus laparoscopic hysterectomy with lymphadenectomy in treatment of endometrial cancer: a case-matched controlled study of the first one hundred twenty two patients. Gynecol Oncol 120:413–418
12. Lin CH, Wei FC, Levin LS et al (1999) Donor-site morbidity comparison between endoscopically assisted and traditional harvest of free latissimus dorsi muscle flap. Plast Reconstr Surg 104: 1070–1077
13. Maxwell GP, McGibbon BM, Hoopes JE (1979) Vascular considerations in the use of a latissimus dorsi myocutaneous flap after a mastectomy with an axillary dissection. Plast Reconstr Surg 64:771–780
14. McCraw JB, Dibbell DG, Carraway JH (1977) Clinical definition of independent myocutaneous vascular territories. Plast Reconstr Surg 60:341–352
15. Miller MJ, Robb GL (1995) Endoscopic technique for free flap harvesting. Clin Plast Surg 22:755–773
16. Pomel C, Missana MC, Lasser P (2002) Endoscopic harvesting of the latissimus dorsi flap in breast reconstructive surgery. Feasibility study and review of the literature. Ann Chir 127: 337–342 [French]
17. Ramakrishnan VV, Southern S, Villafane O (1997) Endoscopic harvest of the latissimus dorsi muscle using the balloon dissection technique. Plast Reconstr Surg 99:899–903; discussion 904–905
18. Ramakrishnan VV, Southern SJ (1997) Endoscopic rectus harvest: a simplified sheath-saving technique. Ann Plast Surg 39:573–577
19. Ramirez OM, Ruas E, Dellon AL (1990) "Components separation" method for closure of abdominal-wall defects: an anatomic and clinical study. Plast Reconstr Surg 86:519–526
20. Schneider WJ, Hill HL Jr, Brown RG (1977) Latissimus dorsi myocutancous flap for breast reconstruction. Br J Plast Surg 30:277–281
21. Seitz IA, Adler N, Odessey E (2009) Latissimus dorsi/rib intercostal perforator myo-osseocutaneous free flap reconstruction in composite defects of the scalp: case series and review of literature. J Reconstr Microsurg 25:559–567
22. Suominen S, Asko-Seljavaara S, von Smitten K et al (1996) Sequelae in the abdominal wall after pedicled or free TRAM flap surgery. Ann Plast Surg 36:629–636
23. Tansini I (1906) Sopra il mio muovo processo di amputazione della mammella. Gazetta Medica Italiana 67:141

Head and Neck 18

Jesse Creed Selber

18.1 Introduction

The oropharynx can be considered anatomically as a somewhat irregularly shaped cylinder. Oropharyngeal cancers, by definition, lie within this cylinder. In order to access and resect a certain subset of these tumors, this cylinder needs to be opened. Traditionally, this has been done either by dividing the mandible and sometimes the lip or by making a pharyngotomy that is sufficiently wide to resect and deliver the tumor. Unfortunately, mandibulotomies and large phayngotomies can result in significant postoperative morbidity and functional compromise (Fig. 18.1). Because of the morbidity involved in some of these more aggressive resections, and the proven efficacy of chemoradiation in the treatment of some oropharyngeal cancer, there was a paradigm shift away from ablative surgery [2, 13]. As long-term follow-up on these "organ-sparing" protocols has begun to take shape, however, significant morbidity and mortality have emerged. In one recent study, chemoradiation therapy was associated with 4 % treatment related death, 6 % osteoradionecrosis, 12 % chronic aspiration, 12 % nonhealing ulcers, and 42 % serious adverse events [5]. And although these protocols are intended to preserve normal anatomy, normal speech and swallowing are far from assured. Studies assessing intermediate- and long-term adverse events following chemotherapy and radiation reveal that patients often experience substantial functional impairment, including persistent swallowing difficulties and dysphonia, xerostomia, diminished vocal ability, and airway compromise with a propensity for aspiration [1, 4, 9, 10].

Transoral robotic surgery (TORS) was developed to resect tumors in the oropharynx without splitting the mandible. TORS has been adopted at multiple other centers and was FDA approved in 2009 [3, 7, 8, 14, 15]. Functional and oncologic outcomes are

J.C. Selber, M.D., M.P.H.
Department of Plastic Surgery – Unit 1488, Anderson Cancer Center,
The University of Texas, M.D., 1400 Pressler St., Houston 77030, TX, USA
e-mail: jcselber@mdanderson.org

P. Liverneaux et al. (eds.), *Telemicrosurgery*,
DOI 10.1007/978-2-8178-0391-3_18, © Springer-Verlag France 2013

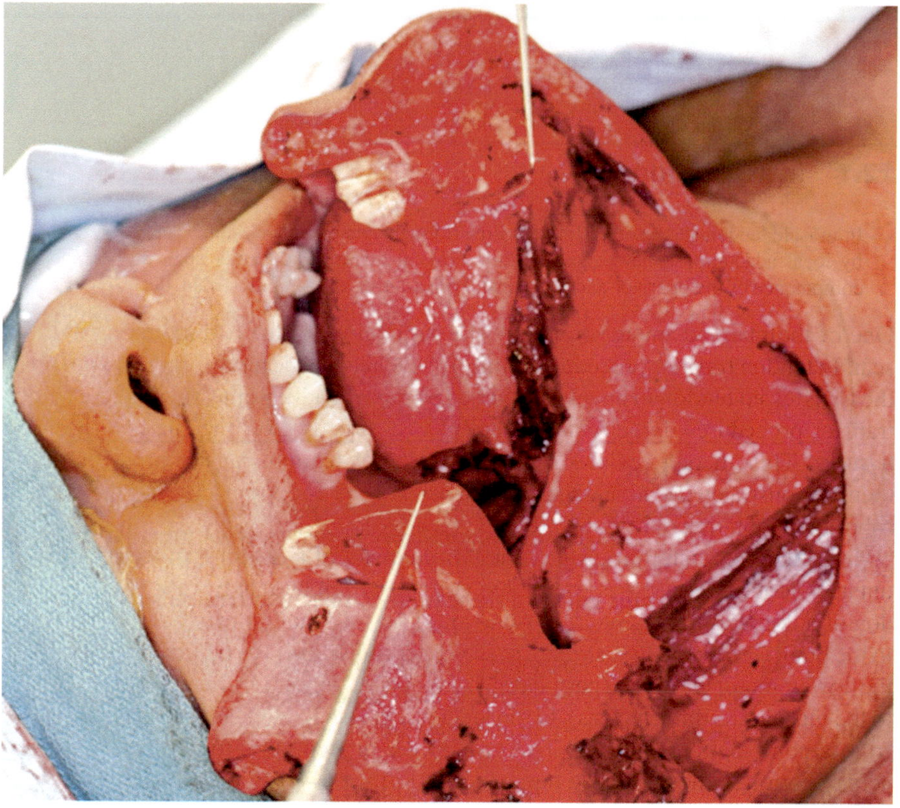

Fig. 18.1 Access to challenging oropharyngeal tumors has traditionally been through a mandibulotomy or wide pharyngotomy approach. Because of the morbidity of these procedures, as well as the proven effectiveness of chemoradiation therapy, there has been a paradigm shift away from ablative surgery. Unfortunately, chemoradiation therapy is also associated with profound morbidity and even mortality

currently being investigated in the setting of prospective clinical trials at the University of Pennsylvania, the Mayo Clinic, Mount Sinai Medical Center, the University of Alabama, and the University of Texas M.D. Anderson Cancer.

Transoral robotic resections can provide the benefits of locoregional control without the morbidity of wide pharyngeal access or high-dose radiation. Many of these tumors can be removed completely transorally. A mouth retractor is used to set the interdental opening; two robotic arms and the endoscope are placed in the mouth, converging on the target pharyngeal anatomy, and the tumor is resected with the surgeon sitting at the robotic console. Occasionally, these tumors are too large for a complete transoral resection, and in these cases a small lateral pharyngotomy can be added for additional exposure.

In its initial use, the standard following TORS resections was that oropharyngeal defects were allowed to heal by secondary intention. This approach was reliable for smaller tumors, but not in cases where a significant anatomic defect is created.

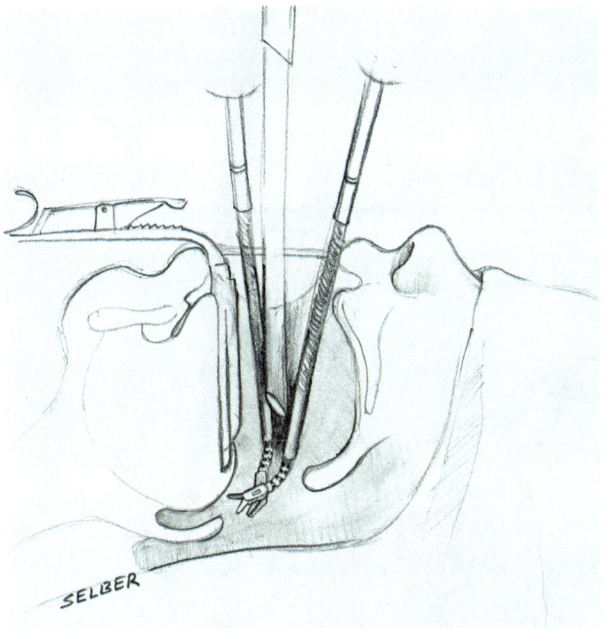

Fig. 18.2 Robotic inset of oropharyngeal reconstructions helps mitigate the space restrictions associated with robotic resections, where the cylinder of the oropharynx remains almost entirely closed. The setup involves a mouth retractor to set the interdental opening. The two robotic arms and endoscope are then placed in the mouth, converging on the target oropharyngeal anatomy

These cases require soft tissue reconstruction. The reconstructive challenge, however, created by these minimally invasive resections is that the cylinder of the oropharynx remains almost entirely closed, severely restricting access to oropharyngeal anatomy. In particular, the anatomic region between the uvula and the epiglottis is very difficult to approach without a mandibulotomy or wide pharyngotomy. For these types of defects, transoral inset of a free flap or local flap using robotic assistance has been shown to be both feasible [11] and effective [12]. By taking this approach, the plastic surgeon can provide the reconstructive support for the head and neck surgeon to remove larger and more complex tumors robotically that would be very difficult to reconstruct through traditional methods.

18.2 Surgical Procedure

18.2.1 Robotic Flap Inset

The setup for the robotic portion is similar for all cases (Fig. 18.2). First, an optical window is created in the mouth. When the tongue base is not involved, a Dingman retractor (other retractors have also been tested for this use and employed clinically [6]) is placed in the mouth to create a stable interdental opening and provide lingual retraction. When reconstruction of the base of tongue is required, the tongue must remain mobile. In these cases, a suture is placed in the tip of the tongue for manipulation, a mouth prop creates the interdental opening, and a cheek retractor is placed to maintain a stable frame (Fig. 18.3).

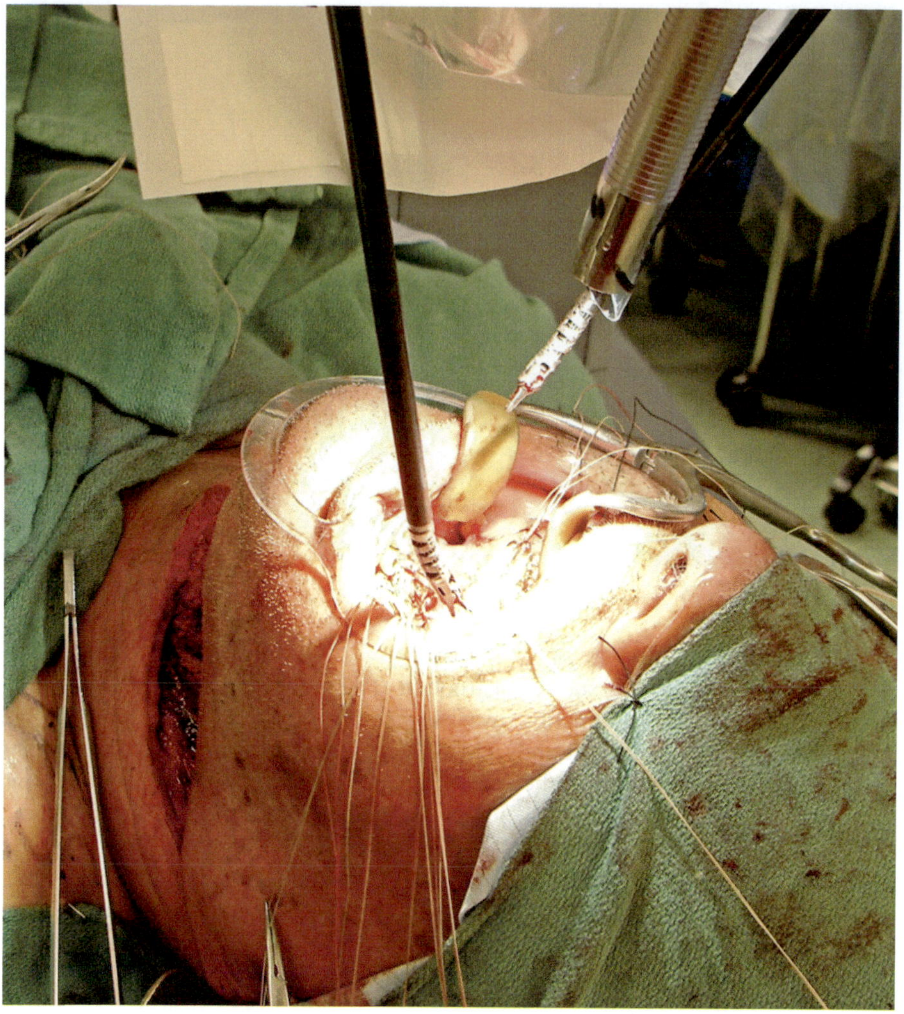

Fig. 18.3 When reconstruction of the base of tongue is required, the tongue must remain mobile. In these cases, a suture is placed in the tip of the tongue for manipulation, a mouth prop creates the interdental opening, and a cheek retractor is placed to maintain a stable frame

The exact location and position of the patient side cart will change depending on the location of the defect. The way the robot is designed, the arms function best when the working area is lined up with the base, and the arms are working back toward it; therefore, when a defect is in the right tonsillar area, the robot should be positioned at 45° to foot of the right side of the bed. When a defect is in the left tonsillar area, 45° from the foot of the left side is preferred. For a central, posterior pharynx, either of these two positions is adequate. In each of these cases, the patient side cart should be against the base of the bed, to bring it as close to the mouth as

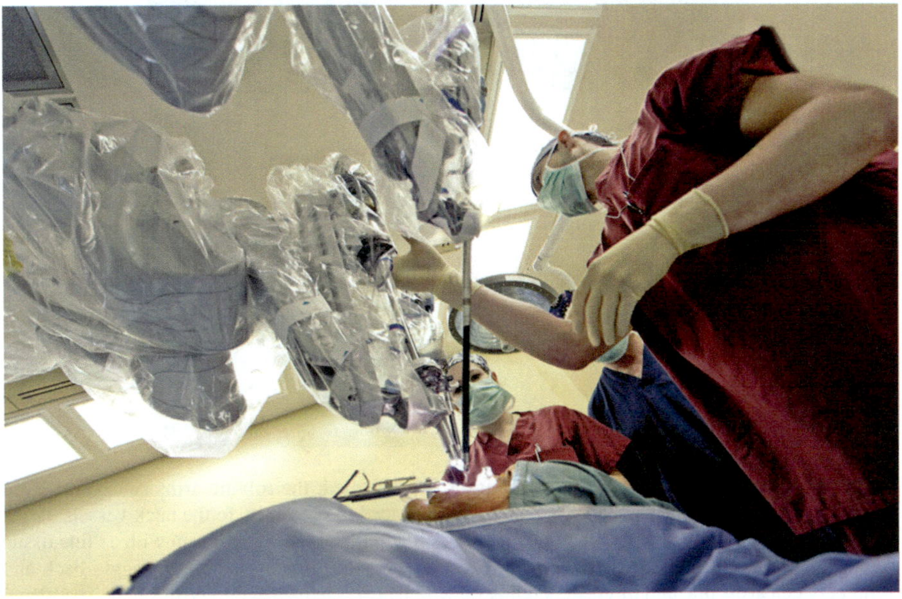

Fig. 18.4 The exact location and position of the patient side cart will change depending on the location of the defect. The way the robot is designed, the arms function best when the working area is lined up with the base and the endoscope, and the arms are working back toward it. The shoulders of the three arms should be angled at 90°, and the arms should form approximately 45° angles with the endoscope

possible. When operating on the palate, bringing the robot in from the head of the bed may work better. No matter which of these approaches is used, the two robotic arms are aligned around a point converging at the target anatomy in the oropharynx. The shoulders of the three arms should be angled at 90°, and the arms should form approximately 45° angles with the endoscope (Fig. 18.4).

After the method of reconstruction is chosen and the flap elevated, inset within the mouth is performed using two 8-mm needle drivers and 4.0 or 3.0 Vicryl suture. Two needle drivers are preferable to a needle driver and grasper because it is sometimes necessary to throw sutures with both robot arms, depending on the angle and location within the oral cavity.

The suture is trimmed to approximately 3 in. in length, in order to avoid extra suture material in the mouth. Interrupted sutures are placed and tied using the robot. Economy of motion is important because small movements at the tips of the instruments correspond to large movements more proximally where excursion of the robotic arms is limited by the area within the mouth retractor. On occasion, when the space is too restricted such as in the glossopharyngeal sulcus, sutures can be placed robotically, taking advantage of the improved visualization, and then tied down blindly by hand.

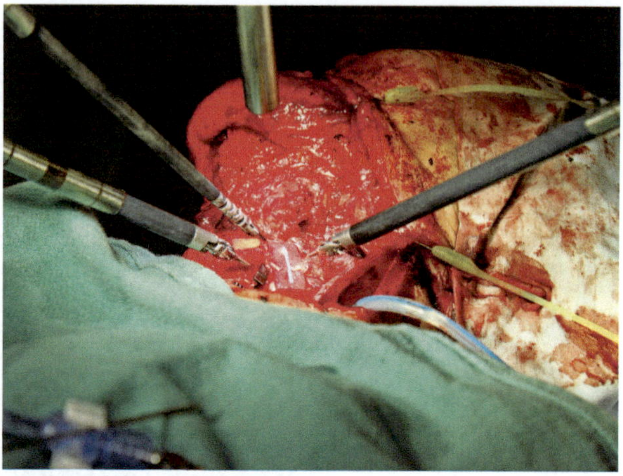

Fig. 18.5 Once the robotic portion of the inset is performed, the robotic arms can be removed from the mouth, instruments changed, and the arms placed in proximity to the neck vessels. Arms one and two are equipped with Black Diamond microneedle driver. A third arm with a "fine tissue forceps" attachment serves as a stationary assistant, and the surgeon is able to toggle back and forth between arms one and three, depending on which arm is being used to position the vessel and which is being used to sew 9.0

18.2.2 Robot-Assisted Microvascular Anastomosis

Once the robotic portion of the inset is performed, the robotic arms can be removed from the mouth, instruments changed, and the arms placed in proximity to the neck vessels (Fig. 18.5). Arms one and two are equipped with Black Diamond® microneedle drivers (Intuitive Surgical™, Sunnyvale, CA, USA), rather than the larger-jawed needle drivers used during the inset. A third arm with a "fine tissue forceps" attachment serves as a stationary assistant, and the surgeon is able to toggle back and forth between arms one and three, depending on which arm is being used to position the vessel and which is being used to sew. 9.0 nylon suture is used for the anastomosis.

There are advantages and disadvantages to robot-assisted microvascular anastomosis. The main advantage is precision. The robot is capable of up to 5–1 motion scaling, meaning the surgeon moves the hand-operated mechanism 5 cm, and the robotic arms respond by moving 1 cm. Another advantage is 100 % tremor elimination. The combination of motion scaling and tremor elimination greatly enhances precision, which is the foundation of microsurgery. Another advantage is surgeon comfort. We often ignored this to our own detriment, but it is very important over the life of a microsurgeon. The robotic console is very ergonomic and comfortable (Fig. 18.6).

The main disadvantage is a lack of haptic or tactile feedback, although I thought this would be a much bigger problem than it has turned out to be. What I have learned is that in microsurgery, much of what we think we feel,

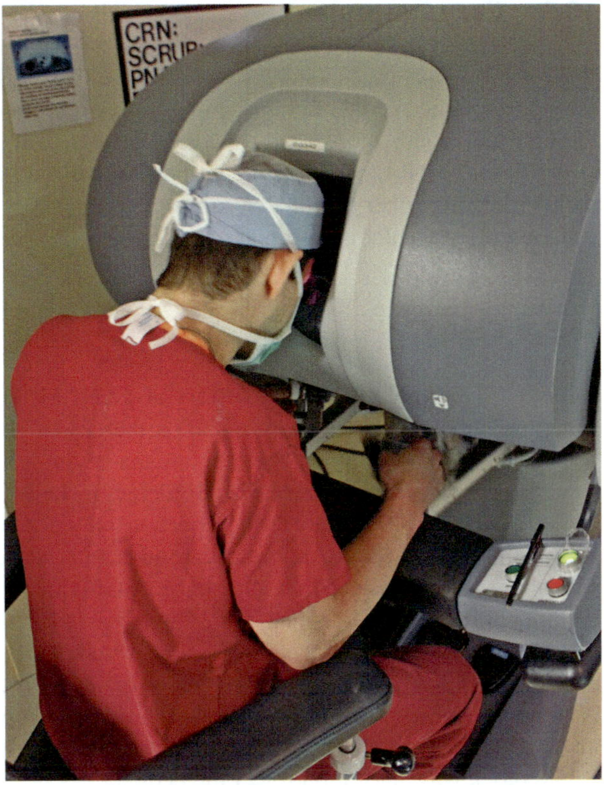

Fig. 18.6 Another advantage is of robotic microsurgery is surgeon comfort. Microsurgeons often ignore this to their own detriment, but it is very important over the duration of a career. The robotic console is very ergonomic and comfortable. There is minimal neck and back strain

we actually see and our brains are supplying the illusion of sensation. That being said, the robot is very strong, and one has to pay close attention to visual cues, particularly when it comes to setting down the knot. It is important to maintain equal slack in both ends of the suture, try to minimize movement of the anastomosis while tying (as this represents a differential in applied tension), and only pull until the air in the knot disappears. These measures minimize vessel trauma. Another disadvantage is the instrumentation. The currently available microinstruments are called Black Diamond® microneedle drivers. These instruments are poorly designed for microsurgery. The tips are too broad and flat, and the surface is coated with diamond dust, which has a tendency to cut the suture. RAMSES helped the company to design instruments more like the ones to which we are accustomed and they are up for FDA approval. Finally, in some systems, the image is low definition. I would recommend use of a 1,080 dpi, high-resolution video system if one is going to endeavor to do microsurgery robotically. This is especially important because, unlike the operating microscope which has optical zoom, the robot is only capable of digital zoom. The consequence is that increasing the magnification past a certain point actually decreases the resolution.

18.3 Case Examples

The following two case examples represent the two ends of the spectrum of applications for robotic reconstructions. For smaller resections, local flaps can be inset through the mouth more easily in the posterior pharyngeal using the robot. For larger defects, the upper pharyngeal portion can be inset robotically through the mouth, the lower pharyngeal area can be inset manually through the pharyngotomy, and the microvascular anastomosis can also be performed robotically.

18.3.1 Case 1

NO is a 74-year-old male with a history of T2 N1 M0 right, tonsillar squamous cell carcinoma treated with primary radiation therapy in 1997. He subsequently developed a T2 N0 M0 squamous cell carcinoma of the left tonsil. He underwent transoral robotic resection of the tumor. His defect included the posterior tonsillar pillar, a portion of the soft palate, and a portion of the posterior pharynx (Fig. 18.7). Although the defect was small, the carotid sheath was exposed and there was concern about velopharyngeal incompetence. A left-sided, inferiorly based facial artery myomucosal flap was planned. The flap extended from the ipsilateral retromolar trigone to the frenulum of the gingivobuccal sulcus (Fig. 18.8). The flap was passed over the third molar and into the defect to reconstruct the posterior tonsillar pillar. A Dingman retractor was used to create an interdental opening and retract the cheeks and tongue. Inset of the flap was performed robotically using 4.0 Vicryl sutures. A bite block was placed to protect the pedicle.

18.3.2 Case 2

RH is a 62-year-old-man with a history of recurrent T3 N1 M0 squamous cell carcinoma of the left posterolateral pharynx following failed radiation treatment in the past (Fig. 18.9). He underwent a combination transoral robotic resection with the addition of a small lateral pharyngotomy and a left neck dissection. Although the pharyngotomy was small (approximately 15 cm^2), a large portion of the pharynx (approximately 50 cm^2) was resected from the epiglottis to the soft palate (Fig. 18.10). A 6 × 9 cm radial forearm flap was harvested (Fig. 18.11). The upper pharyngeal component was inset robotically. The remainder of the inset was completed through the pharyngotomy. The patient side cart, which was already in position from the

Fig. 18.7 This 74-year-old male with a T2 N0 M0 squamous cell carcinoma of the left tonsil underwent transoral robotic resection of the tumor. His defect included the posterior tonsillar pillar, a portion of the soft palate, and a portion of the posterior pharynx. The defect and specimen are shown here

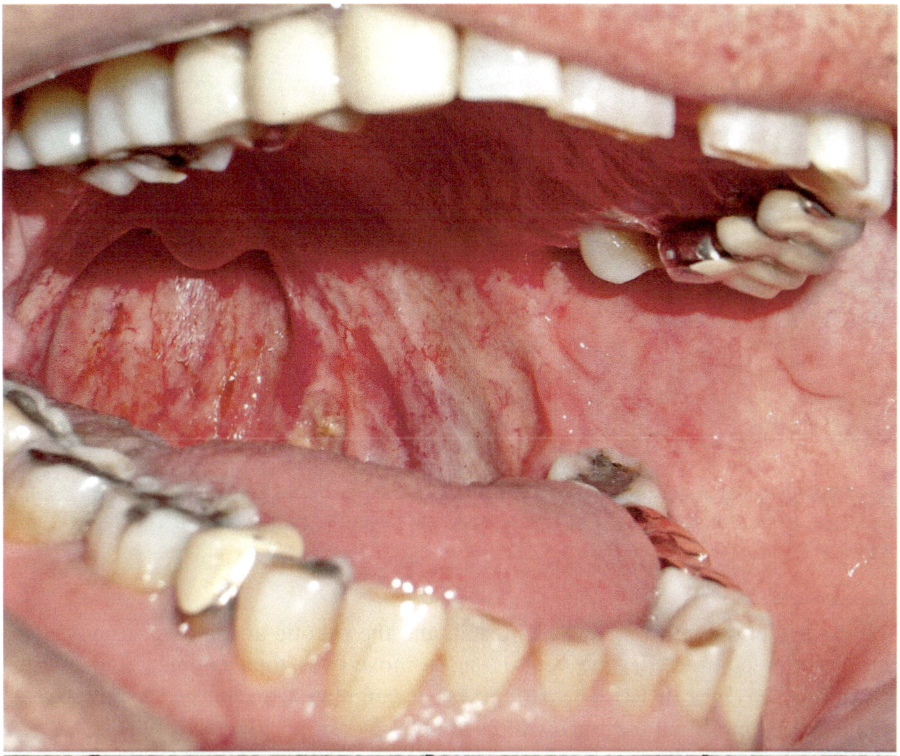

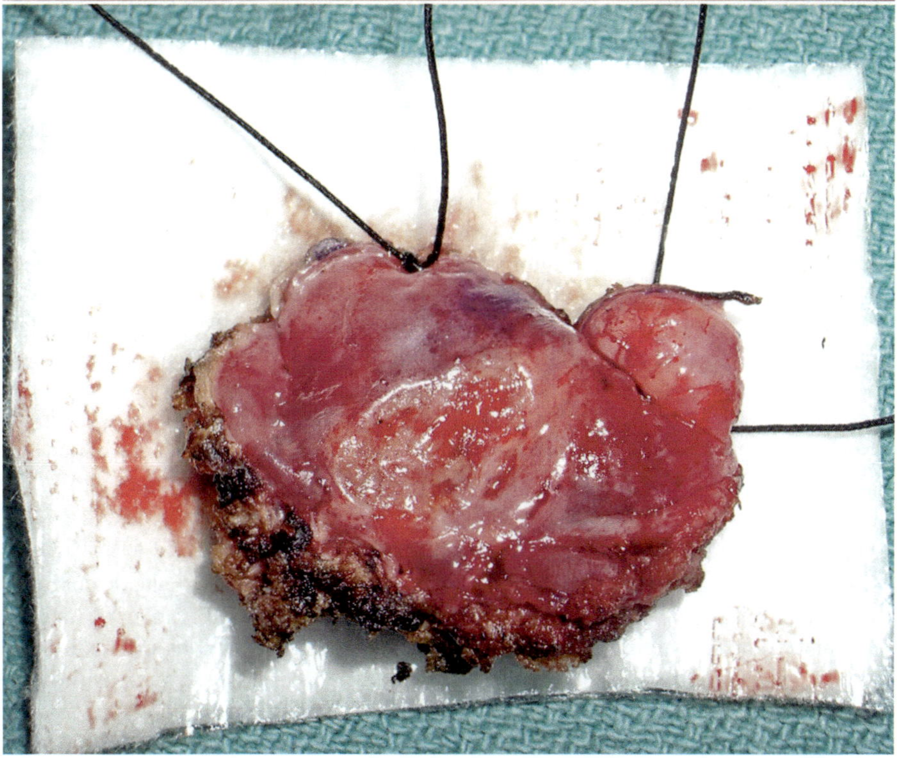

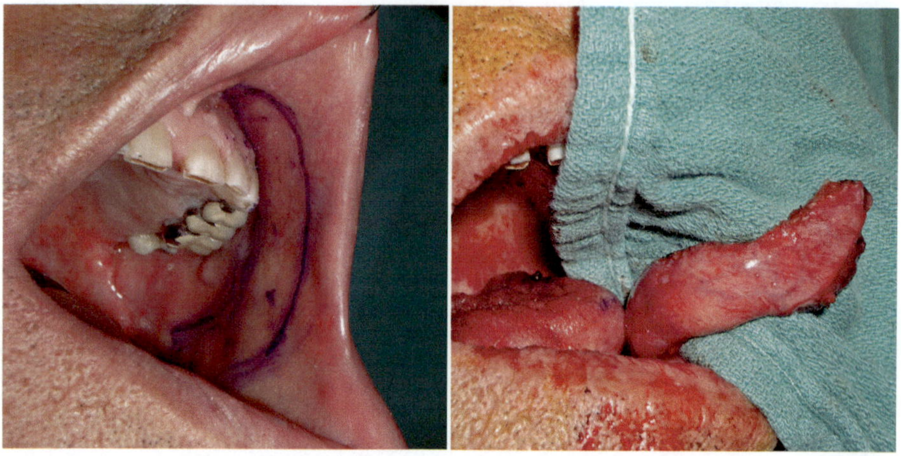

Fig. 18.8 A facial artery myomucosal flap was elevated, as shown here. It was passed back into the defect to restore velopharyngeal competence and cover the carotid sheath. The flap was inset robotically

robotic resection and inset, was adjusted, and the robotic arterial anastomosis was successfully completed. The venous anastomosis was then coupled under loupe magnification (Fig. 18.12). The patient was decannulated, discharged within a week, and passed a modified barium swallow study 3 weeks postoperatively (Fig. 18.13). His speech and swallowing are normal, and he is tolerating a regular diet independent of tube feeds (Fig. 18.14).

18.4 Discussion

Approaches to oropharyngeal tumors have traditionally involved relatively morbid procedures through an approach involving a mandibulotomy or wide pharyngotomy. As a result of a series of data demonstrating the efficacy of chemoradiation for head and neck cancer, there was a shift away from ablative surgery. The combination of complications from high-dose chemoradiation therapy, the development of minimally invasive approaches to head and neck surgery, and the emergence of younger patients with HPV, P-16 positive tumors have caused the pendulum to begin to swing back toward ablative surgical treatment, particularly with the advent of transoral robotic resections. Minimally invasive resections have opened the door for many tumors to be treated surgically, with lower morbidity. Functional and oncologic outcomes have been good, and some patients receiving TORS resections do not even require tracheostomy.

These minimally invasive resections have moved reconstructive plastic surgeons to engage minimally invasive reconstructive techniques. The range of defects encountered in this setting are quite broad. Some smaller resections, particularly in the base of tongue, require no reconstruction at all. Other defects, such as those in

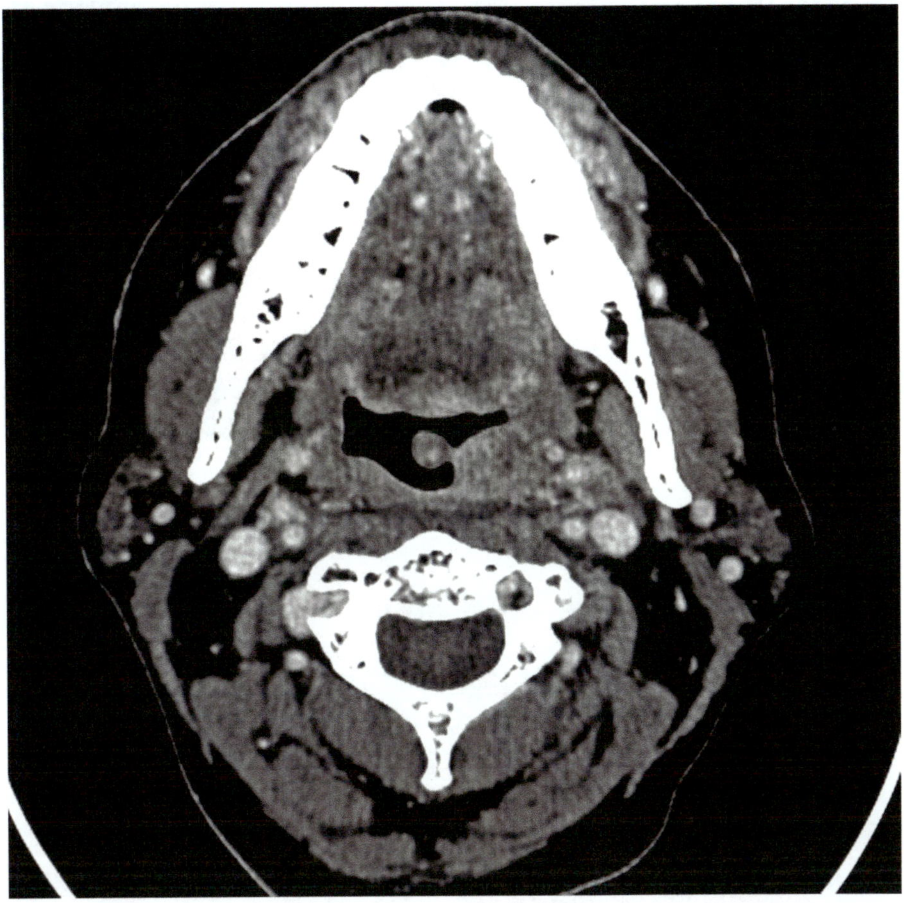

Fig. 18.9 This is the CT of a 62-year-old man with a history of recurrent T3 N1 M0 squamous cell carcinoma of the left posterolateral pharynx following failed radiation treatment. The encroachment of the tumor on the pharynx is apparent

the tonsillar areas and partial soft palate defects, create exposure of the carotid sheath and the potential for velopharyngeal incompetence. These defects can be treated with facial artery myomucosal flaps, buccal rotation flaps, and pharyngeal flaps. Defects resulting from larger tumor resections are often topographically complex and may extend from the tip of the tongue all the way to the epiglottis, involving a significant pharyngeal component and a pharyngotomy. These types of defects usually require a combination of transoral robotic inset and manual inset through the pharyngotomy defect. In these cases, it is important to note that although a pharyngotomy has been created, this is much smaller than the wide pharyngotomies traditionally required to access such tumors, because access to the upper pharynx is achieved robotically rather than through the neck.

Fig. 18.10 Although the pharyngotomy is quite small, the defect itself extends well into the oropharynx. This poses a difficult access problem which can be solved by performing the oropharyngeal portion of the inset robotically

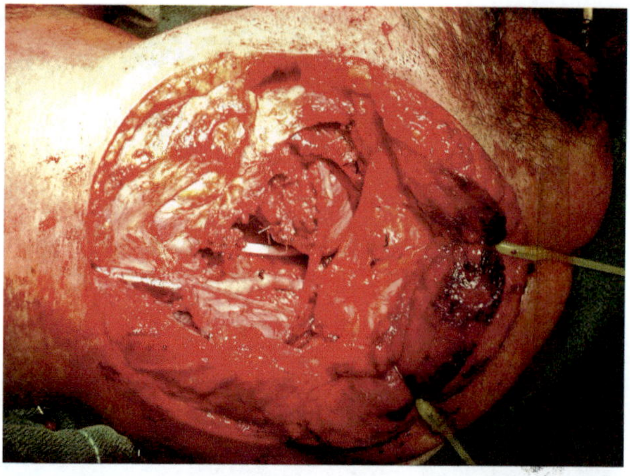

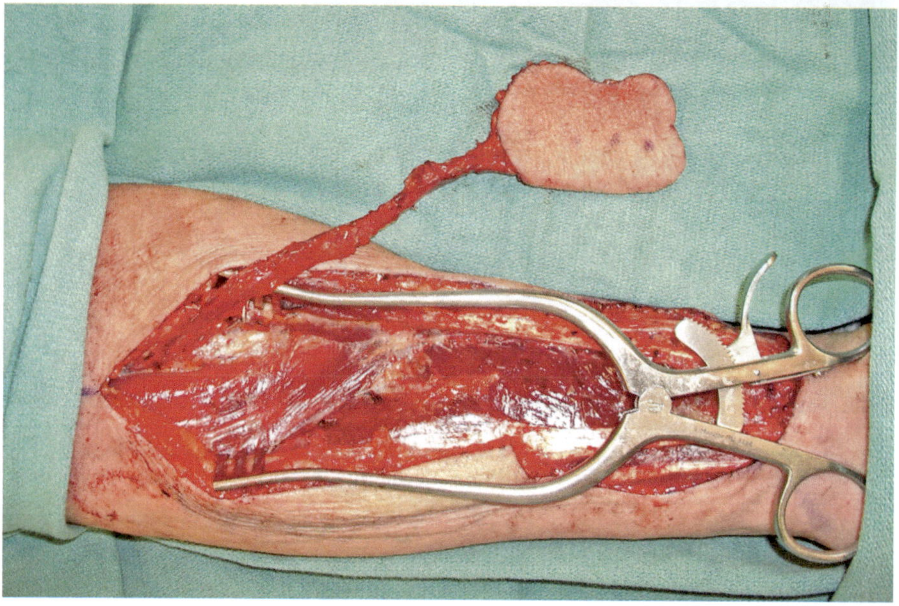

Fig. 18.11 A radial forearm flap is designed from a template that fits the oropharyngeal defect

Finally, robotic microvascular anastomosis is a burgeoning application. Microvascular anastomoses can be challenging in certain head and neck cases. The facial artery is the most common recipient artery but can be difficult to use. It is found passing under the hypoglossal nerve and beneath the digastric sling, often

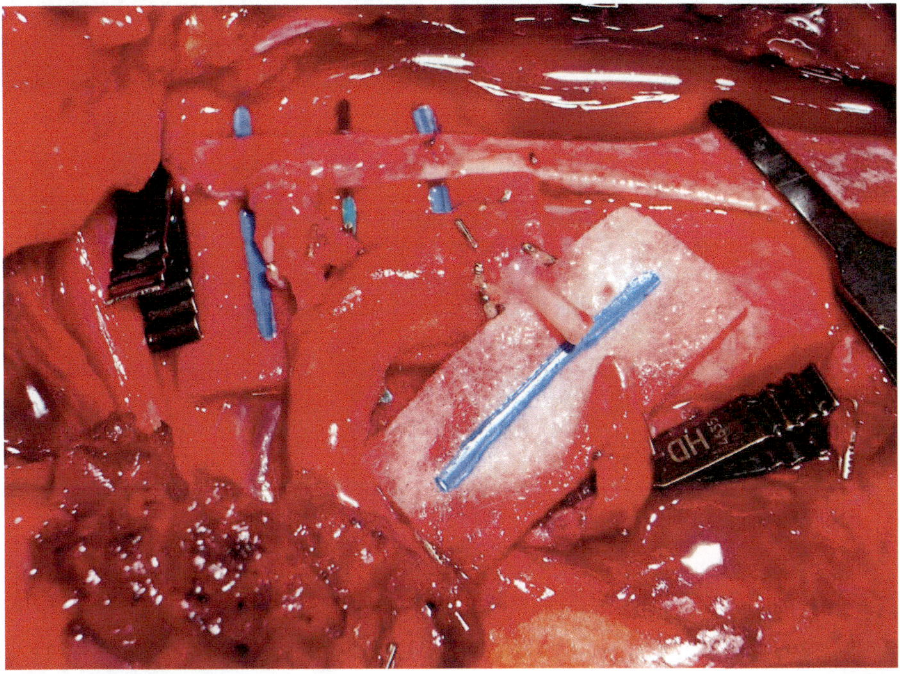

Fig. 18.12 The venous pedicle is anastomosed to a side branch of the internal jugular vein under loupe magnification. The radial and, in this case, the superior thyroid arteries are cleaned under loupe magnification and set up over a background to be anastomosed robotically

high under the body of the mandible. If a tracheostomy and ventilator tubing is also connected, the space available to perform the anastomosis may be restricted. The robot's precision and visualization in confined spaces make it well suited for anastomoses in such cases. The available instrumentation is small enough to handle 9.0 needles, there is 100 % tremor elimination, and scaling can be adjusted to reduce movements 5–1 for higher precision. Although these techniques are not perfect, advances in robotic technology may make robotic microvascular surgery much more common.

Conclusion

Minimally invasive resections are of great benefit to patients and represent a true advance in the field of head and neck surgery. If such techniques are to be become the standard, reconstructive methods must keep pace. The techniques described in this chapter allow the plastic surgeon to actively collaborate in a movement toward less morbid procedures for patients with head and neck cancer.

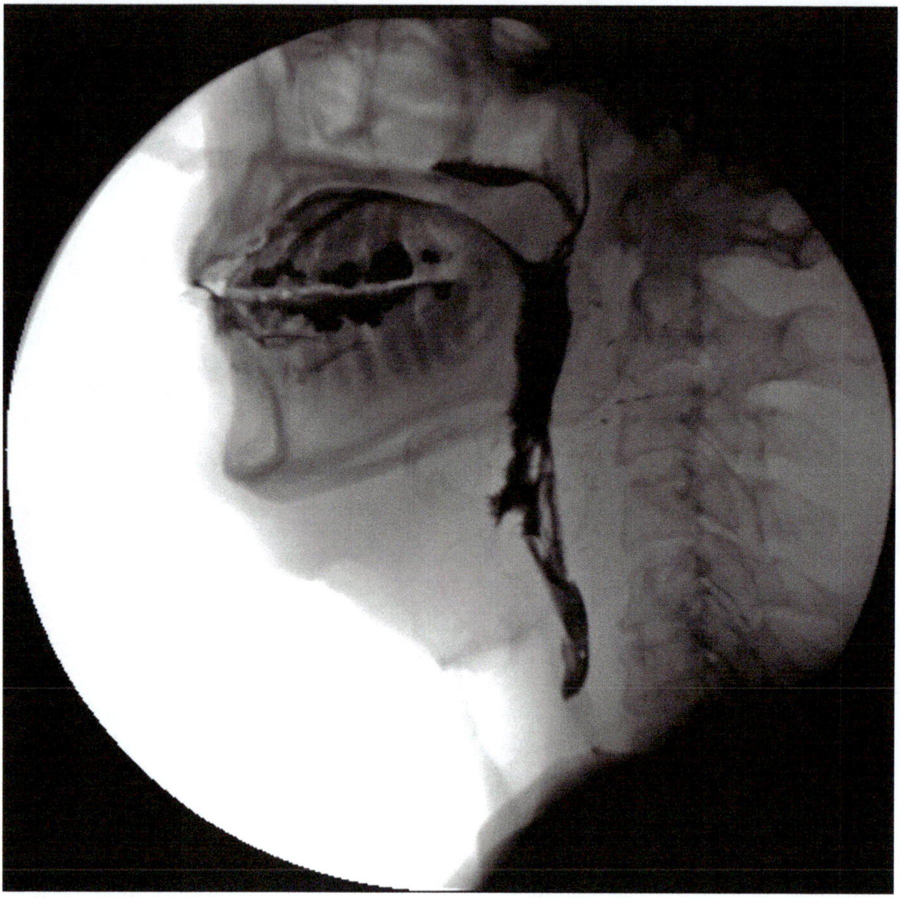

Fig. 18.13 A modified barium swallow demonstrates no leak and no aspiration. There is mild nasopharyngeal regurgitation as a result of some soft palate resection

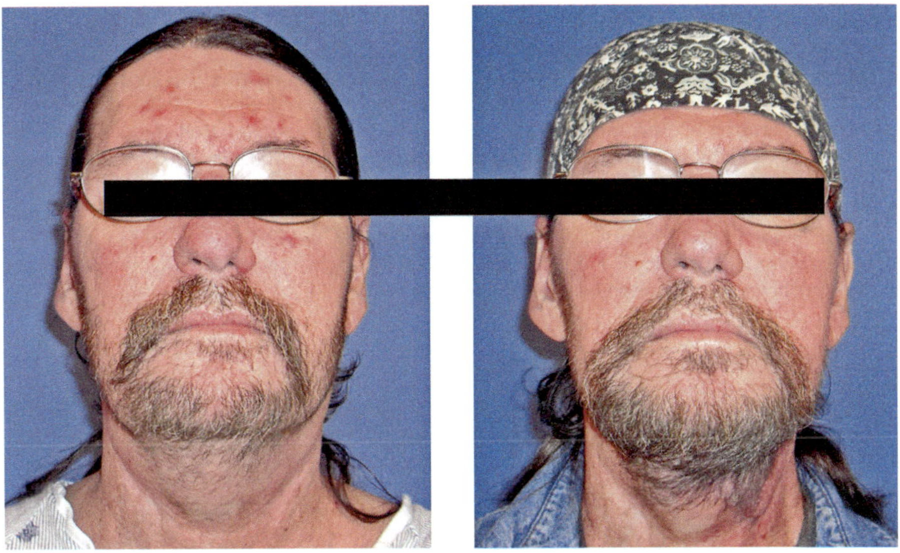

Fig. 18.14 Besides a small amount of weight loss in the face, the patient looks very similar in preoperative and postoperative photos, in spite of having a very large operation. This excellent cosmetic result is because a mandibulotomy and labiotomy were avoided by using the robot for both resection and reconstruction

References

1. Campbell BH, Spinelly K, Marbella AM et al (2004) Aspiration, weight loss, and quality of life in head and neck survivors. Arch Otolaryngol Head Neck Surg 130:1100–1103
2. Forastiere AA, Goepfert H, Maor M et al (2003) Concurrent chemotherapy and radiotherapy for organ preservation in advanced laryngeal cancer. N Engl J Med 349:2091–2098
3. Genden EM, Desai S, Sung CK (2009) Transoral robotic surgery for the management of head and neck cancer: a preliminary experience. Head Neck 31:283–289
4. Kotz T, Costello R, Li Y, Posner MR (2004) Swallowing dysfunction after chemoradiation for advanced squamous cell carcinoma of the head and neck. Head Neck 26:365–372
5. Machtay M, Rosenthal DI, Hershock D, Penn Cancer Center Clinical Trials Group et al (2002) Organ preservation therapy using induction plus concurrent chemoradiation for advanced resectable oropharyngeal carcinoma: a University of Pennsylvania Phase II Trial. J Clin Oncol 20:3964–3971
6. O'Malley BW, Weinstein GS, Snyder W et al (2006) Trans-oral robotic surgery (TORS) for base of tongue neoplasms. Laryngoscope 116:1465–1472
7. Ozer E, Waltonen J (2008) Trans-oral robotic nasopharyngectomy: a novel approach for nasopharyngeal lesions. Laryngoscope 118:1613–1616
8. Park YM, Lee WJ, Lee JG, Chi EC et al (2009) Trans-oral robotic surgery (TORS) in laryngeal and hypopharyngeal cancer. J Laparoendosc Adv Surg Tech A 19:361–368
9. Rademaker AW, Vonesh EF, Logemann JA et al (2003) Eating ability in head and neck cancer patients after treatment with chemoradiation: a 12-month follow-up study accounting for dropout. Head Neck 25:1034–1041
10. Roh JL, Kim AY, Cho MJ (2005) Xerostomia following radiotherapy of the head and neck. J Clin Oncol 23:3016–3023

11. Selber JC (2010) Trans oral robotic reconstruction of oropharyngeal defects: a case series. Plast Reconstr Surg 126:1978–1987
12. Selber JC, Robb G, Serletti JM et al (2010) Transoral robotic free flap reconstruction of oropharyngeal defects: a preclinical investigation. Plast Reconstr Surg 125:896–900
13. The Department of Veterans Affairs Laryngeal Cancer Study Group (1991) Induction chemotherapy plus radiation compared with surgery plus radiation in patients with advanced laryngeal cancer. N Engl J Med 324:1685–1690
14. Weinstein GS, O'Malley BW Jr, Snyder W et al (2007) Trans-oral robotic surgery: radical tonsillectomy. Arch Otolaryngol Head Neck Surg 133:1220–1226
15. Weinstein GS, O'Malley BW Jr, Snyder W et al (2007) Trans-oral robotic surgery: supraglottic partial laryngectomy. Ann Otol Rhinol Laryngol 116:19–23

Urology

19

Sijo Joseph Parekattil

19.1 Introduction

Since the advent of the operating microscope for microsurgery in 1975 [31], there has been a steady increase in the use of such technology in the operative management of male infertility and chronic testicular or groin pain [3, 7, 12, 17, 18, 20, 27, 29, 31–33]. Greater patency and fertility rates of vasovasostomy performed with the operating microscope [21] were achieved. More recently, microscopic spermatic cord neurolysis has demonstrated applicability for the treatment of chronic groin and testicular pain [16, 19]. These microsurgical techniques require varying degrees of microsurgical skills and can be technically demanding. Improved visualization with magnification in a stable ergonomic platform would be of great benefit. To this end, robotic-assisted microsurgery (telemicrosurgery) has been utilized in a wide array of microsurgical procedures [4, 5, 9, 13, 24].

This chapter covers current evaluations of various robotic microsurgical applications for male infertility and patients with chronic testicular or groin pain.

19.2 Setup in Robotic-Assisted Microsurgery in Urology

19.2.1 New Robotic Surgical Platform

Intuitive Surgical™ (Sunnyvale, CA, USA) now offers an enhanced 4-arm da Vinci type Si® robotic system with high-definition digital visual magnification that allows for greater magnification than the standard robotic system (up to 10–15×). The enhanced magnification capability allows the surgeon to position the camera 6–7 cm away from the operative field to avoid any local tissue effects from the heat emitted

S.J. Parekattil, M.D.
Department of Urology, Winter Haven Hospital, University of Florida,
200 Avenue F. N.E., Winter Haven 33881, FL, USA
e-mail: sijo.parekattil@winterhavenhospital.org

P. Liverneaux et al. (eds.), *Telemicrosurgery*,
DOI 10.1007/978-2-8178-0391-3_19, © Springer-Verlag France 2013

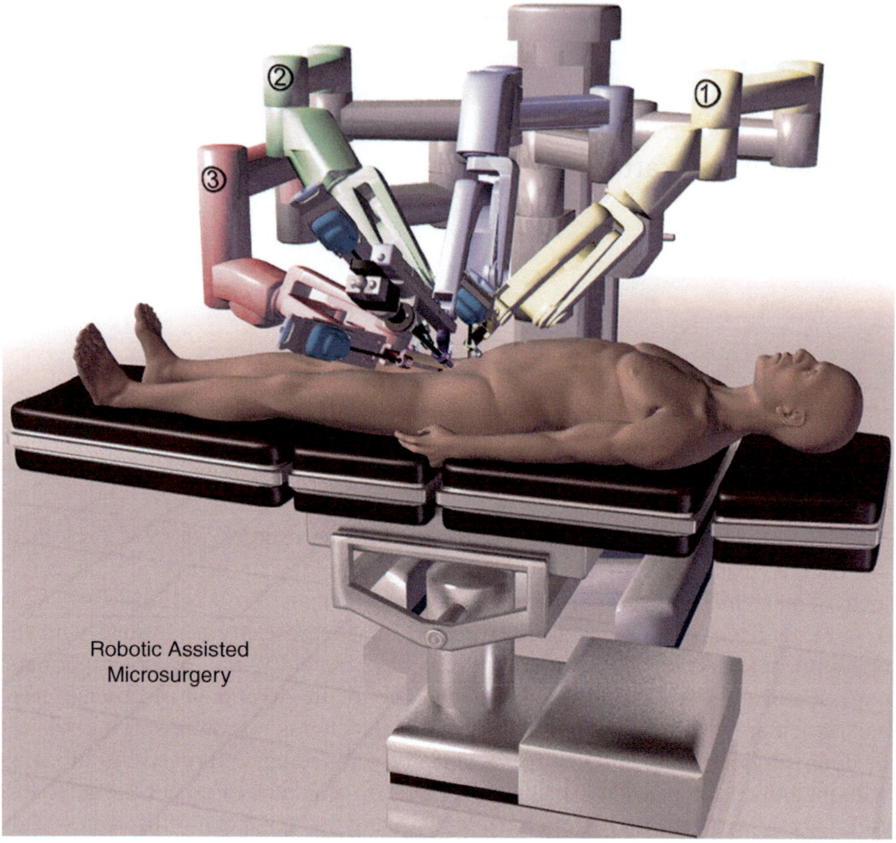

Fig. 19.1 Robotic platform positioning for microsurgical cases (Sijo Joseph Parekattil)

from the camera lighting (this was a problem with the older system, where the camera had to be placed within 2–3 cm of the operative field for microsurgery). This new system allows greater range of motion and better microsurgical instrument handling. The additional fourth arm has improved range of motion and positioning capabilities to provide the microsurgeon with one additional tool during procedures.

19.2.2 Operative Setup

The robot is positioned from the right side of the patient for microsurgical cases (Fig. 19.1). A large high-definition monitor at the foot of the patient allows the surgical assistant and the surgical nursing team to easily visualize the operative field and prepare instruments and suture for each step of the procedure. We also utilize the VITOM® (Karl Storz™, Inc., Tuttlingen, Germany) camera lens system with the TilePro™ robot console software system to view up to three video screens simultaneously (see the chapter on robotic instruments for a detailed description and images).

19.2.3 Patient Positioning

The patient is placed in the supine position. The table is placed level (there is no Trendelenberg). The robot is brought in from the right side of the patient after skin incisions are made and the operative tissues exposed. The arms of the patient may be placed alongside (gently wrapped in the draw sheets) or apart on arm boards with adequate padding to prevent any nerve compression injuries. Sequential compression devices are placed on the lower extremities to reduce the risk of deep venous thrombus formation. A foley catheter is generally not utilized; however, if the procedure lasts more than 2 h, the patient is usually straight catheterized at the end of the procedure to drain the bladder (before recovering the patient from anesthesia).

19.2.4 Trocar Configuration

The robot is positioned after skin incisions are made and operative tissues are exposed. The robot is used to perform the microsurgical components of the procedure. Since this is an open case, the trocars are loaded only to allow the instruments to function and to stabilize their movements outside the patient's body. It is important to advance the instruments at least 4–5 cm beyond the tip of the trocar when positioning the robotic arms to optimize range of motion. The fourth robotic arm may be placed lateral to the left robotic arm to minimize instrument clashes. The zero-degree camera lens is used to optimize the visual field during procedures.

19.3 Some Robotic Microsurgical Applications

19.3.1 Robotic-Assisted Microscopic Vasectomy Reversal (RAVV)

A number of groups have developed robotic-assisted techniques to perform RAVV in animal and ex vivo human models (Fig. 19.2) [14, 15, 25, 26, 28]. Some studies suggest robotic-assisted reversal may have advantages over microsurgical reversal in terms of ease of performing the procedure and improved patency rates [25, 26]. A few groups have actually performed human robotic-assisted vasovasostomies using the initial da Vinci® robotic system (Intuitive Surgical, Sunnyvale, CA) [11]. These efforts have been recently confirmed in human RAVV cases performed using the new da Vinci SI® system [22, 23].

A recent prospective control study of robotic versus pure microsurgical vasectomy reversal in 123 vasectomy reversal cases performed from August 2007 to April 2011 by a single fellowship-trained microsurgeon was performed. The primary end point was operative duration. The secondary end point was total motile sperm count at 2, 5, 9, and 12 months postoperatively. Case breakdown was as such: 48 cases bilateral RAVV, 30 cases robotic-assisted vasoepididymostomy (RAVE) on at least one side, 28 cases bilateral microsurgical vasovasostomy (MVV), and 17 cases microsurgical vasoepididymostomy (MVE) on at least one side. Selection of approach

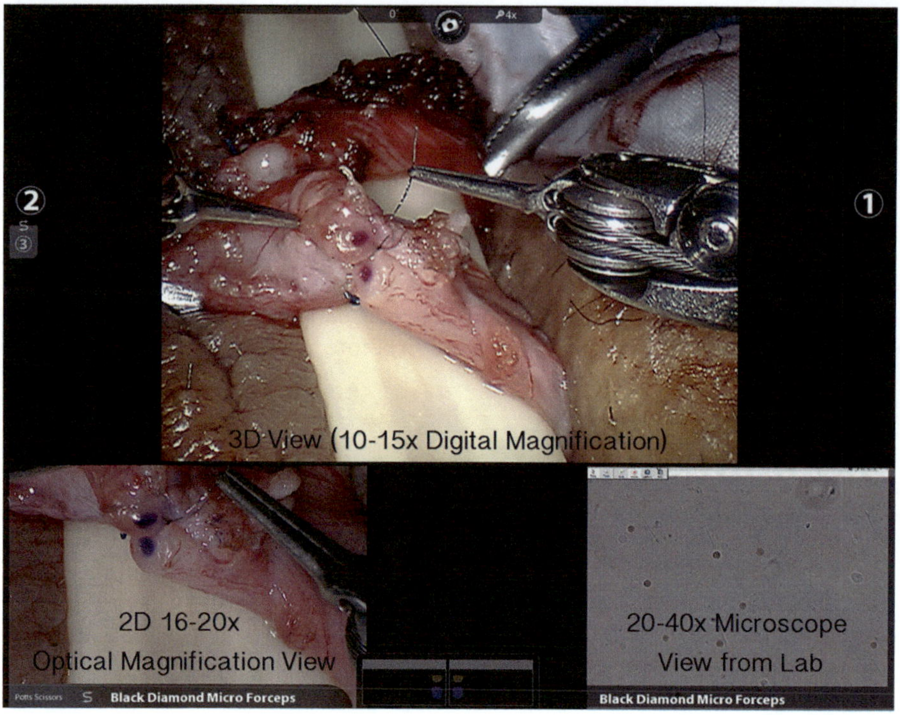

Fig. 19.2 Robotic-assisted microsurgical vasovasostomy (RAVV). The right robotic arm is equipped with Black Diamond® microforceps. The left robotic arm is equipped with Black Diamond® microforceps. The fourth robotic arm is equipped with Potts scissors. The assistant uses an irrigation via 10-cc syringe with 18-gauge angiocatheter (Sijo Joseph Parekattil)

(robotic vs. pure microscopic) was based on patient choice. Preoperative patient characteristics were similar in both groups. The same suture materials and suturing techniques (2-layer 10-0 and 9-0 nylon anastomosis for vasovasostomy; 10-0 nylon double-armed longitudinal intussusception technique for vasoepididymostomy) were used in both approaches.

Mean clinical follow-up was 14 months (range 2–37 months). patency was achieved in the RAVV cases and 80 % in MVV (>1 million sperm/high-power field). Median operative duration was significantly decreased in RAVV at 90 min (40–180) compared to MVV at 120 min (60–180), $p=0.0001$. RAVE at 120 min (60–180) was significantly faster than MVE at 161 min (120–240), $p=0.001$. Mean postoperative total motile sperm counts were not significantly higher in RAVV/RAVE versus MVV/MVE, but the rate of postoperative sperm count recovery was significantly greater in RAVV/RAVE. The improved efficiency and eliminated need for a skilled assistant in RAVV/RAVE have reduced the cost of this reversal procedure to less than the regional average cost for MVV/MVE. The total out-of-pocket cost for the patient for a robotic-assisted vasectomy reversal at our institution now is $5,500.

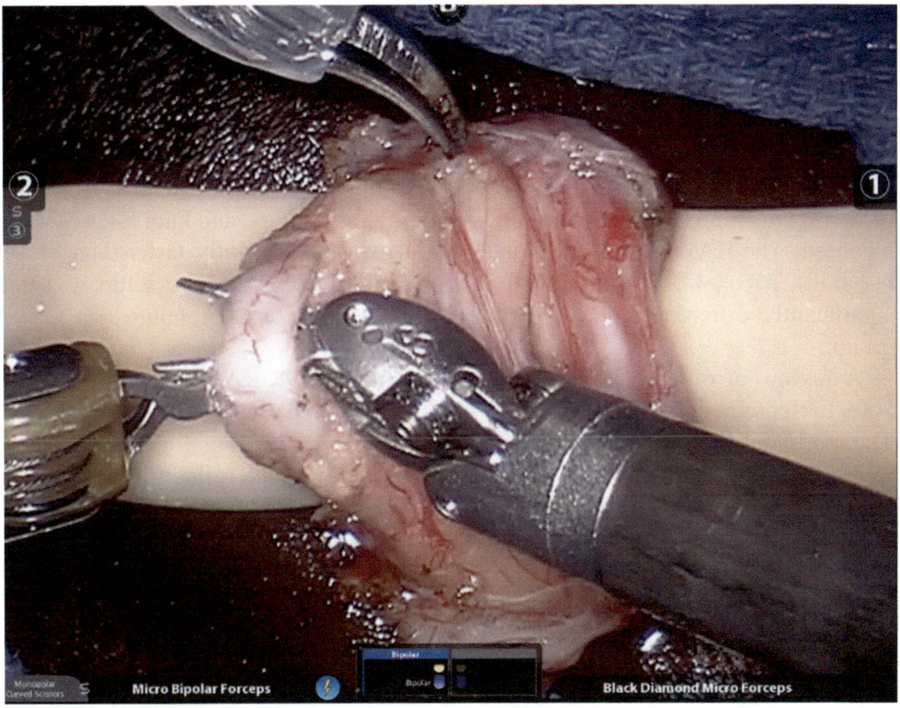

Fig. 19.3 Robotic-assisted microsurgical subinguinal varicocelectomy (RAVx). The right robotic arm is equipped with Black Diamond® microforceps. The left robotic arm is equipped with micro-bipolar forceps. The fourth robotic arm is equipped with curved monopolar scissors. The assistant uses an irrigation via 10-cc syringe with 18-gauge angiocatheter and passes 3-0 silk suture ties (1.5″ length). Robotic micro Doppler probe (Vascular Technology™, Inc, Nashua, NH, USA) is utilized for intraop arterial identification (Sijo Joseph Parekattil)

The use of robot assistance in microsurgical vasovasostomy and vasoepididymostomy may have potential benefit over MVV and MVE with regard to decreasing operative duration and improving the rate of recovery of postoperative total motile sperm counts. Further evaluation and longer follow-up is needed to assess its clinical potential and the true cost-benefit ratio.

19.3.2 Robotic-Assisted Microscopic Varicocelectomy (RAVx)

Although reports of robotic-assisted laparoscopic intraabdominal varicocelectomy have been published [10], there are a number of publications that suggest that microscopic subinguinal varicocelectomy (MVx) may provide superior outcomes compared to intraabdominal varicocelectomy [1, 2, 6, 8]. Shu et al. were the first to publish on robotic-assisted microsurgical subinguinal varicocelectomy (RAVx) (Fig. 19.3) [30]. They compared standard microsurgical to robotic-assisted varicocelectomy and found that the robotic approach provided advantages in terms of slightly decreasing operative duration and complete elimination of surgeon tremor.

To further explore these findings, we performed a prospective randomized control trial of MVx to RAVx in a canine varicocele model by a fellowship-trained microsurgeon. The surgeon performed cord dissection and ligation of three veins with 3-0 silk ties. Twelve canine varicocelectomies were randomized into two arms of six: MVV versus RAVx. Procedure duration, vessel injury, and knot failures were recorded. The RAVx mean duration (9.5 min) was significantly faster than MVV (12 min), $p=0.04$. The duration for robot setup and microscope setup was not significantly different. There were no vessel injuries or knot failures in either group.

A review of our prospective clinical database of 97 RAVx cases from June 2008 to September 2010 (median follow-up 11 months: range 1–27) is as follows. The median duration per side was 30 min (10–80). Indications for the procedure were the presence of a grade two or three varicocele and the following conditions: 10 with azoospermia, 42 with oligospermia, and 49 with testicular pain (with or without oligospermia and failed all other conservative treatment options). Three-month follow-up was available for 81 patients: 75 % with oligospermia had a significant improvement in sperm count or motility, and one with azoospermia was converted to oligospermia. For testicular pain, 92 % had complete resolution of pain (targeted neurolysis of the spermatic cord had been performed in addition to varicocelectomy). One recurrence or persistence of a varicocele occurred (by physical and ultrasound exam), one patient developed a small postoperative hydrocele, and two patients had small postoperative scrotal hematomas (treated conservatively). The fourth robotic arm allowed the surgeon to control one additional instrument during the cases decreasing reliance on the microsurgical assistant. The fourth arm also enabled the surgeon to perform real-time intraoperative Doppler mapping of the testicular arteries while dissecting the veins with the other arms if needed.

Robotic-assisted microsurgical subinguinal varicocelectomy appears to be safe, feasible, and efficient. The preliminary human results appear promising. Further evaluation and comparative effectiveness studies are warranted.

19.3.3 Robotic-Assisted Testicular Sperm Extraction (ROTESE)

Testicular sperm extraction (TESE) is a microsurgical procedure utilized in men with nonobstructive azoospermia. Our goal was to assess if robotic surgery (da Vinci Si™ with high-definition magnification system) may offer any advantages to microsurgical TESE procedures. A robotic technique was developed and compared to standard micro TESE and percutaneous needle lavage (PNL) techniques.

A robotic technique for TESE was developed. A prospective randomized blinded trial utilizing 18 canine testicles and 6 surgeons of varying experience level was designed to compare 3 TESE techniques: ROTESE (Fig. 19.4), open

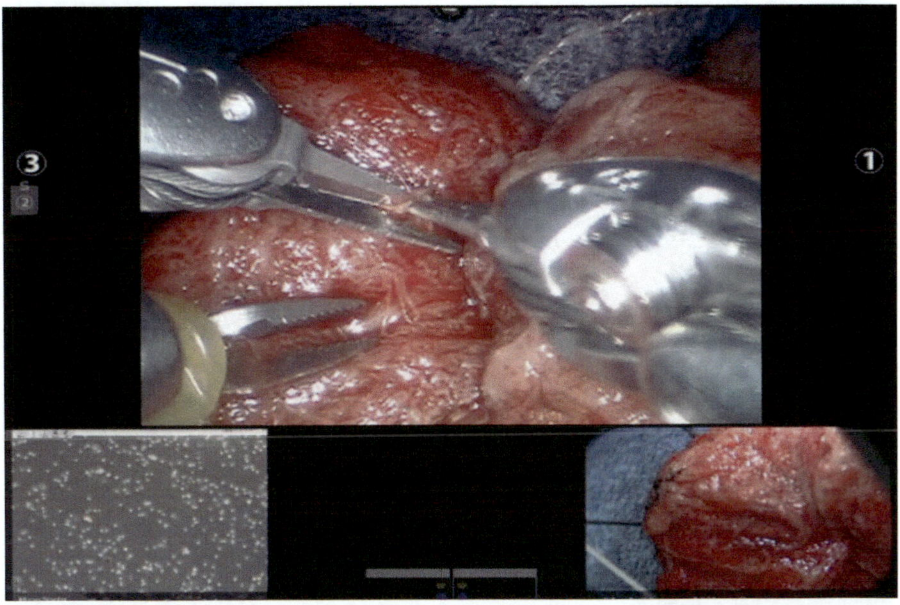

Fig. 19.4 Robotic-assisted microsurgical testicular sperm extraction (ROTESE). The right robotic arm is equipped with Black Diamond® microforceps. The left robotic arm is equipped with micro-bipolar forceps. The fourth robotic arm is equipped with curved monopolar scissors. The assistant uses an irrigation via 10-cc syringe with 18-gauge angiocatheter and brings glass slides next to field for specimen collection (Sijo Joseph Parekattil)

micro TESE, and PNL. Three different color dye spots were injected into all testicles in random locations. The time to detection of these spots within the testicles and number of these spots identified using each technique was analyzed. Our first ten human ROTESE cases performed from July 2007 to March 2011 were also reviewed.

Overall color spot detection accuracy in the animal study for ROTESE, TESE, and PNL was 89, 94 and 39 %, respectively. The difference in ROTESE and TESE accuracy was not statistically significant ($p=0.56$). However, both ROTESE and TESE were significantly more accurate than PNL ($p<0.01$). ROTESE was significantly longer in duration in novice surgeons compared to TESE. However, in experienced robotic surgeons, there was no difference in duration.

ROTESE in all ten human patients was completed successfully without any complications. The first case was 4 h in duration, the second was 3 h in duration, and the most recent case only took us approximately 1 h. Subjectively, ROTESE did appear to make tissue handling and dissection slightly easier and ergonomic compared to open TESE. The use of the TilePro™ triview software at the surgeon console was very helpful since it allowed the image from a Nikon dissecting microscope used by the embryologist/andrologist to dissect through the testicular tissue to be simultaneously accessible to the microsurgeon, thus improving operative efficiency when looking for sperm.

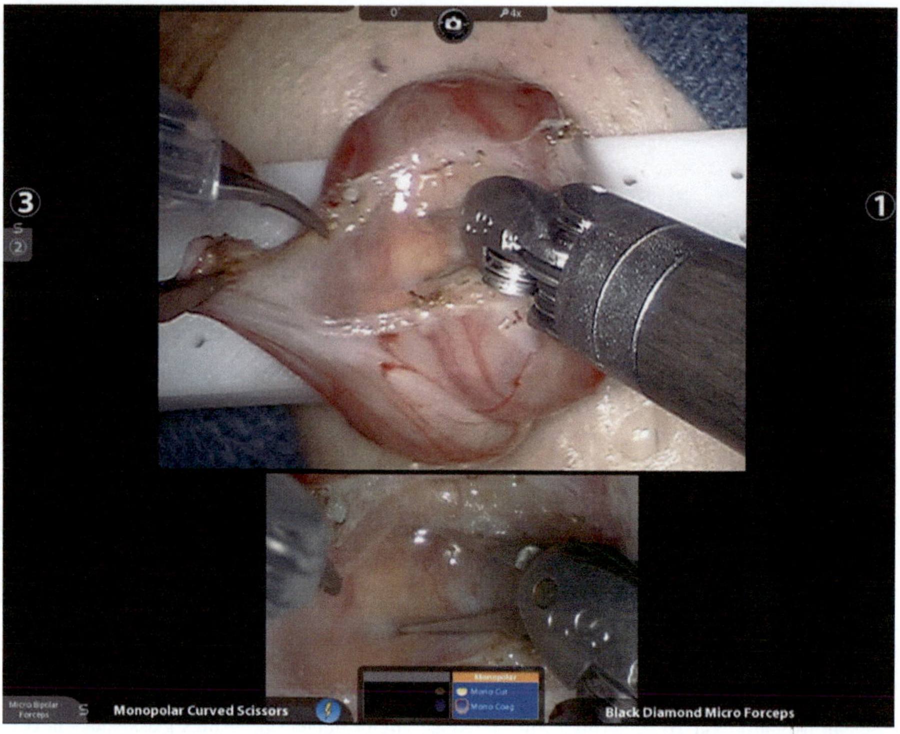

Fig. 19.5 Robotic-assisted microsurgical denervation of the spermatic cord (RMDSC). The right robotic arm is equipped with Black Diamond® microforceps. The left robotic arm is equipped with microbipolar forceps. The fourth robotic arm is equipped with curved monopolar scissors. The assistant uses an irrigation via 10-cc syringe with 18-gauge angiocatheter. Robotic micro Doppler probe (Vascular Technology, Inc.) is utilized for intraop arterial identification (Sijo Joseph Parekattil)

In the animal model, ROTESE appears to be just as effective as open TESE. Both ROTESE and open TESE appear to be superior to PNL in detection accuracy. ROTESE may have a learning curve in novice surgeons and robotic experience seems to be beneficial. ROTESE appears to be a safe technique in humans from our preliminary experience. Further evaluation and analysis is needed to assess its potential.

19.3.4 Robotic-Assisted Microscopic Denervation of the Spermatic Cord (RMDSC)

Recent studies by Levine et al. [16] and Oliveira et al. [19] have shown that microscopic denervation of the spermatic cord is an effective treatment option for men with chronic testicular pain. Our group has been developing a robotic-assisted microsurgical approach for the denervation of the spermatic cord (RMDSC) to assess if there may be any potential benefit over the standard microscopic technique (Fig. 19.5).

A review of our initial 313 RMDSC cases from October 2008 to June 2011 was performed (median follow-up of 13 months – range 1–32). Selection criteria for patients were as such: chronic testicular pain (>6 months), failed standard pain management treatments, and negative urologic workup. A robotic-assisted subinguinal, inguinal, or intraabdominal approach was utilized based on the location of pain. Pain was assessed utilizing a standardized validated questionnaire tool (PIQ-6). The median operative duration was 15 min (5–150). The fourth robotic arm allowed the surgeon to control one additional instrument leading to less reliance on the microsurgical assistant.

Postoperatively, 75 % (234) patients had complete resolution of pain and an additional 10 % (31) had a 50 % or greater decrease in pain. RMDSC was successful in eliminating testicular and or groin pain for a number of possible etiologies: postvasectomy pain syndrome (PVPS), postinguinal hernia pain, sports hernia or groin trauma pain, chronic epididymitis or idiopathic pain, varicocele pain, postrobotic prostatectomy groin or testicular pain, postnephrectomy or donor nephrectomy groin or testicular pain, postpelvic radiation or brachytherapy groin or testicular pain, and fibromyalgia groin pain.

19.3.5 Robotic Single Port or Abdominal Microsurgical Denervation for Phantom Groin Pain After Orchiectomy or Persistent Orchialgia After Denervation of the Spermatic Cord (RAND)

Chronic groin pain can be debilitating for patients. Microsurgical subinguinal denervation of the spermatic cord (MDSC) is a treatment option for this pain. However, there are limited further options for patients who fail this treatment or who have phantom pain after orchiectomy. Our goal was to develop a single port and abdominal robotic microsurgical denervation technique to ligate the genitofemoral and inferior hypogastric nerves fibers within the abdomen above the internal inguinal ring (Figs. 19.6 and 19.7).

We performed a prospective study of patients with chronic groin pain who had either failed previous MDSC or had phantom pain after orchiectomy. Primary end point was impact of pain on quality of life (PIQ-6 pain impact questionnaire from RAND) and secondary end point was operative robotic duration. PIQ-6 scores were collected preop and at 1, 3, 6, and 12 months postop.

We completed 30 cases (5 single port) from June 2009 to September 2010. Elimination of pain occurred in 60 % (18 cases) and a greater than 50 % reduction in pain occurred in an additional 13 % (4 cases) within 1 month postop. Two of the failures were patients that had pain elimination for 6 months, but then pain returned thereafter. Median OR duration was 10 min (5–30). There were three complications: one postop scrotal hematoma that resolved with conservative measures, one patient had pain at one of the port sites, and one patient had pain that shifted from the groin to the leg.

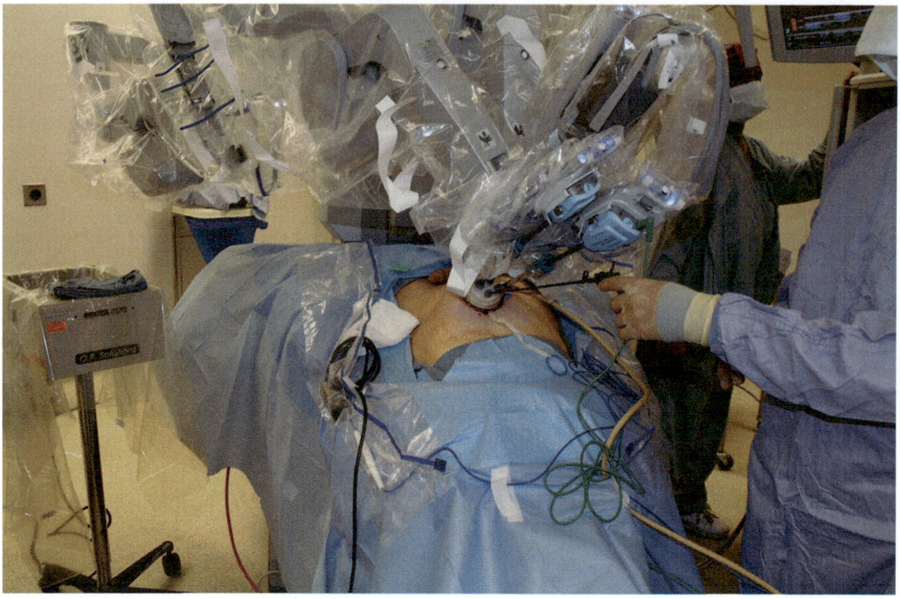

Fig. 19.6 Robotic-assisted abdominal microsurgical denervation (RAND) – external robot setup (Sijo Joseph Parekattil)

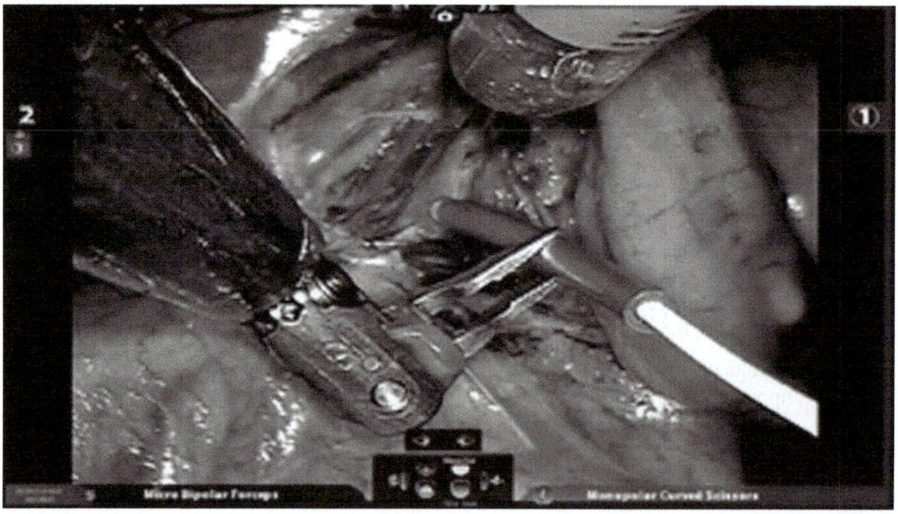

Fig. 19.7 Robotic-assisted abdominal microsurgical denervation (RAND) – intraoperative setup. The right robotic arm is equipped with curved monopolar scissors. The left robotic arm is equipped with microbipolar forceps. Robotic micro Doppler probe (Vascular Technology, Inc.) is utilized for intraop arterial identification (Sijo Joseph Parekattil)

Single port and abdominal robotic microsurgical denervation appears to be an option for treatment in this difficult patient population. Further follow-up and evaluation is warranted.

Conclusions

The use of robot assistance during microsurgical procedures is expanding. The application of this technology in other microsurgery fields apart from urology is also expanding, such as at ophthalmology, hand and nerve surgery, and plastics and reconstructive microsurgery. The advantages of a stable microsurgical platform, ergonomic surgeon instrument controls, elimination of tremor, and magnified immersive 3D vision are all intuitively apparent. Further comparative effectiveness studies are ongoing and will be forthcoming on the true applicability of this new surgical platform. However, the preliminary results so far are quite impressive.

References

1. Al-Kandari AM et al (2007) Comparison of outcomes of different varicocelectomy techniques: open inguinal, laparoscopic, and subinguinal microscopic varicocelectomy: a randomized clinical trial. Urology 69:417–420
2. Al-Said S et al (2008) Varicocelectomy for male infertility: a comparative study of open, laparoscopic and microsurgical approaches. J Urol 180:266–270
3. Berger RE (1998) Triangulation end-to-side vasoepididymostomy. J Urol 159(6):1951–1953
4. Bourla DH et al (2008) Feasability study of intraocular robotic surgery with the Da Vinci surgical system. Retina 28:154–158
5. Casale P (2008) Robotic pediatric urology. Expert Rev Med Devices 5:59–64
6. Cayan S, Shavakhabov S, Kadioglu A (2009) Treatment of palpable varicocele in infertile men: a meta-analysis to define the best technique. J Androl 30:33–40
7. Chan PT, Li PS, Goldstein M (2003) Microsurgical vasoepididymostomy: a prospective randomized study of 3 intussusception techniques in rats. J Urol 169:1924–1929
8. Chen XF et al (2009) Comparative analysis of three different surgical approaches to varicocelectomy. Zhonghua Nan Ke Xue 15:413–416
9. Colombo JR Jr et al (2007) Robotic assisted radical prostatectomy: surgical techniques and outcomes. Int Braz J Urol 33:803–809
10. Corcione F et al (2005) Advantages and limits of robotic-assisted laparoscopic surgery: preliminary experience. Surg Endosc 19:117–119
11. Fleming C (2004) Robotic-assisted vasovasostomy. Urol Clin North Am 31:769–772
12. Fogdestam I, Fall M (1983) Microsurgical end-to-end and end-to-side epididymovasostomy to correct occlusive azoospermia. Scand J Plast Reconstr Surg 17:137–140
13. Guru KA et al (2007) Robotic-assisted radical cystectomy versus open radical cystectomy: assessment of postoperative pain. Can J Urol 14:3753–3756
14. Kuang W et al (2004) Initial evaluation of robotic technology for microsurgical vasovasostomy. J Urol 171:300–303
15. Kuang W et al (2005) Robotic-assisted vasovasostomy: a two-layer technique in an animal model. Urology 65:811–814
16. Levine LA (2008) Microsurgical denervation of the spermatic cord. J Sex Med 5:526–529

17. Marmar JL (2000) Modified vasoepididymostomy with simultaneous double needle placement, tubulotomy and tubular invagination. J Urol 163:483–486
18. Marmar JL, Kim Y (1994) Subinguinal microsurgical varicocelectomy: a technical critique and statistical analysis of semen and pregnancy data. J Urol 152:1127–1132
19. Oliveira RG et al (2009) Microsurgical testicular denervation for the treatment of chronic testicular pain initial results. Clinics (Sao Paulo) 64:393–396
20. Owen ER (2002) Microsurgical vasovasostomy: a reliable vasectomy reversal. J Urol 167:1205
21. Owen ER (1977) Microsurgical vasovasostomy: a reliable vasectomy reversal. Aust N Z J Surg 47:305–309
22. Parekattil SJ, Cohen M, Vieweg J (2009) Human robotic assisted bilateral vasoepididymostomy and vasovasostomy procedures: initial safety and efficacy trial. Proc SPIE 7161:71611L
23. Parekattil SJ, Moran ME (2010) Robotic instrumentation: evolution and microsurgical applications. Indian J Urol 26:395–403
24. Rodriguez E, Chitwood WR Jr (2008) Minimally invasive, robotic cardiac surgery. Ann Thorac Surg 85:357–358
25. Schiff J, Li PS, Goldstein M (2004) Robotic microsurgical vasovasostomy and vasoepididymostomy: a prospective randomized study in a rat model. J Urol 171:1720–1725
26. Schiff J, Li PS, Goldstein M (2005) Robotic microsurgical vasovasostomy and vasoepididymostomy in rats. Int J Med Robot 1:122–126
27. Schlegel PN (1999) Testicular sperm extraction: microdissection improves sperm yield with minimal tissue excision. Hum Reprod 14:131–135
28. Schoor RA, Ross L, Niederberger C (2003) Robotic assisted microsurgical vasal reconstruction in a model system. World J Urol 21:48–49
29. Schultheiss D, Denil J (2002) History of the microscope and development of microsurgery: a revolution for reproductive tract surgery. Andrologia 34:234–241
30. Shu T, Taghechian S, Wang R (2008) Initial experience with robotic-assisted varicocelectomy. Asian J Androl 10:146–148
31. Silber SJ (1975) Microsurgery in clinical urology. Urology 6:150–153
32. Silber SJ (1978) Microscopic vasoepididymostomy: specific microanastomosis to the epididymal tubule. Fertil Steril 30:565–571
33. Thomas AJ Jr (1987) Vasoepididymostomy. Urol Clin North Am 14:527–538

Part V

Perspectives

Supermicrosurgery

20

Takeshi Todokoro and Isao Koshima

20.1 Introduction

Microsurgery of free flaps was developed by Harii, Daniel, and Taylor in 1973 [1, 2] and initially involved the use of a groin flap. Since then, many kinds of free flaps have been developed for microsurgery. The vessels supplying these flaps are small and have a diameter of approximately 1 mm or more.

Koshima introduced perforator flaps in microsurgery [3] during the second stage of development of microsurgery. The merits of using these flaps are that they render the surgery less invasive (muscle and other portions that are harvested for other flaps can be preserved) and can be more suitable for the recipient site as they provide the surgeon with flexibility and multiple choices for donor tissue. While using these flaps, smaller vessels, which are branches of main vessels, need to be accurately detected; however, the vessels used for anastomosis are the same as those used for classic flaps.

Some microsurgeons have developed the skills to anastomose very small vessels. This technique is called "supermicrosurgery" and is defined as anastomosis of vessels that have a diameter of less than 0.5 mm. This technique enables unique operations that seemed impossible earlier, such as fingertip replantation (Fig. 20.1), true perforator flaps [4], and lymphaticovenular anastomosis (LVA) [6] (Figs. 20.2 and 20.3). Supermicrosurgery is an ideal technique in this regard but is very difficult to perform.

20.2 Difficulties in Performing Supermicrosurgery

Performing supermicrosurgery is difficult because of mechanical, technical, and environmental problems related with the small diameter of vessels. These vessels have very thin and soft walls. Therefore, after the vessel is cut, its cut edge closes

T. Todokoro, M.D. (✉) • I. Koshima, M.D., Ph.D.
Department of Plastic and Reconstructive Surgery, The University of Tokyo,
7-3-1, Hongo, Bunkyo-ku, Tokyo, 113-8656, Japan
e-mail: takebou0320@yahoo.co.jp

P. Liverneaux et al. (eds.), *Telemicrosurgery*,
DOI 10.1007/978-2-8178-0391-3_20, © Springer-Verlag France 2013

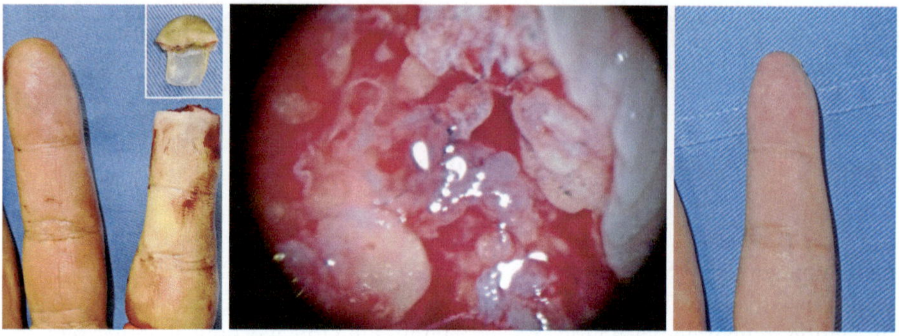

Fig. 20.1 Photographs showing fingertip replantation. *Left*: A palmar view of amputated index fingertip. *Middle*: Arterial anastomosis (the diameters of arteries are 0.3 and 0.45 mm) view under microscope at 20×. *Right*: 6-month follow-up result after reconstruction

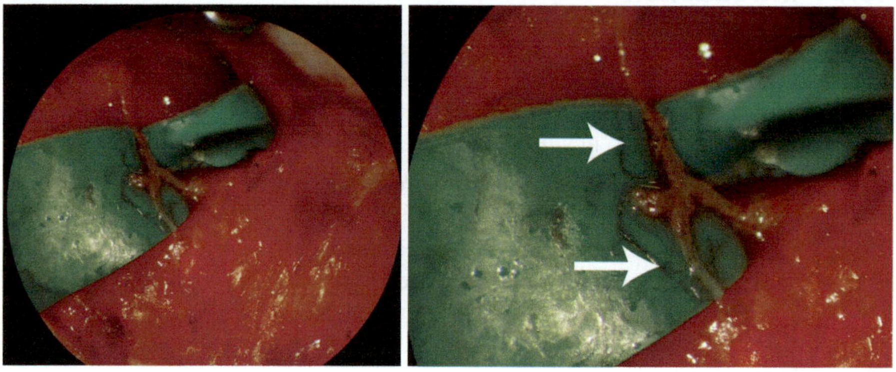

Fig. 20.2 The typical views of LVA. *Left*: A view under microscope at 20×. *Right*: Magnified on computer (*each arrow shows LVA*)

completely, and the intimal edge is often covered with adventitia. Visualizing the inner side of the vessel wall, which faces the lumen, is not difficult, but the inner side can be visualized only for a short period because the walls are soft and cling to each other quickly. In microsurgery, holding the vessel wall from the inner side by using forceps is an essential procedure. However, in supermicrosurgery, it is not possible to insert forceps inside the lumen because of the small diameter of the vessel. Therefore, operators have to penetrate the vessel by using a needle, which is also very small and fragile, without holding the vessel wall from the inner side. The magnification provided by the conventional microscope is not sufficient for supermicrosurgery. Most standard microscopes provide a maximum magnification of 20×. The tubular structure of smaller vessels cannot be seen clearly even at this maximum magnification. When increased magnification is used, operator tremor is more noticeable. This interferes with the very fine aspects of the operation, especially at the stage that the needle is passed through the vessel wall. New techniques

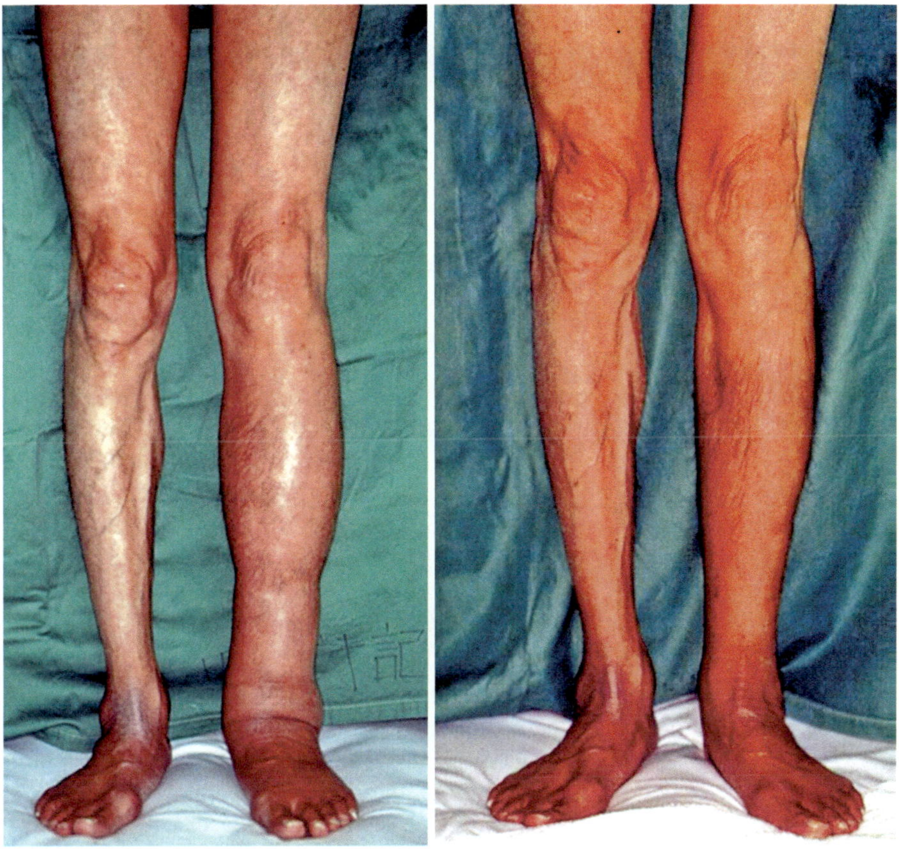

Fig. 20.3 Photographs showing lower extremity lymph edema. *Left*: Preoperative view. *Right*: After performing LVA

and instruments have been invented to overcome these problems, but sufficient progress has not yet been made in this regard.

20.3 Telesupermicrosurgery: The Future Vision of Supermicrosurgery

Telesurgery is used in many fields of surgery and is preferred to traditional surgery in certain fields. Telesurgery is currently not used widely for microsurgery, but the feasibility of telemicrosurgery is being studied. Telesupermicrosurgery may become easier to perform than supermicrosurgery. It has some great advantages that cannot be achieved using manual supermicrosurgery.

One of these is view direction control. The direction of the two vessels that are to be anastomosed is an important factor affecting the ease of anastomosis. In conventional microsurgery, the choice of the vessel from which anastomosis is initiated

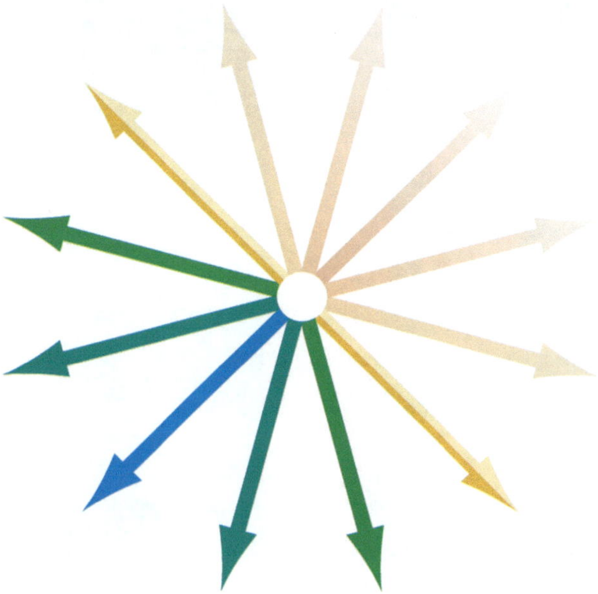

Fig. 20.4 Needle moving direction at microsurgery. *Blue*: easiest direction. *Red*: most difficult direction

has little effect on the results. Therefore, the needle can be moved by almost 180° (Fig. 20.4). In contrast, since the conditions for anastomosis often differ between the vessels during supermicrosurgery, the vessel from which anastomosis is initiated affects ease of performance. Therefore, the needle can be moved in all directions (Fig. 20.5). In telesupermicrosurgery, the field of view can be rotated [5]. Thus, operators can select their consistent and comfortable direction for beginning the anastomosis each time they perform telesupermicrosurgery. Moreover, it is possible to use the mirror view instead of reversing the needle.

Additional advantages of telemicrosurgery are realized through the use of advanced optics. The surgeon benefits from enhancements in magnification and stereoscopic 3D image capture. Limited magnification is obtained with the microscopes commonly used, and only a single image is observed through the eye lens. In supermicrosurgery, greater magnification and quicker image changing between high- and low-power fields are required. In telesupermicrosurgery, increased magnification can be easily achieved using digital zooming because an indirect image is obtained. Using this technology, two images can be reflected in one screen at the same time (Fig. 20.6), similar to that observed with the surgical loupe.

The state of currently available standard manual microsurgical instrumentation confers a limitation to the surgeon. To achieve breakthroughs, finer, more accurate performance and devices are required. Technological advancements in instrumentation for telesupermicrosurgery will improve the facility of performing ultrafine intricate procedures. The surgeon further benefits from the multijoint movement and 6° of freedom associated with the robotic arms and the precision provided by the demultiplication phenomenon described previously in this text.

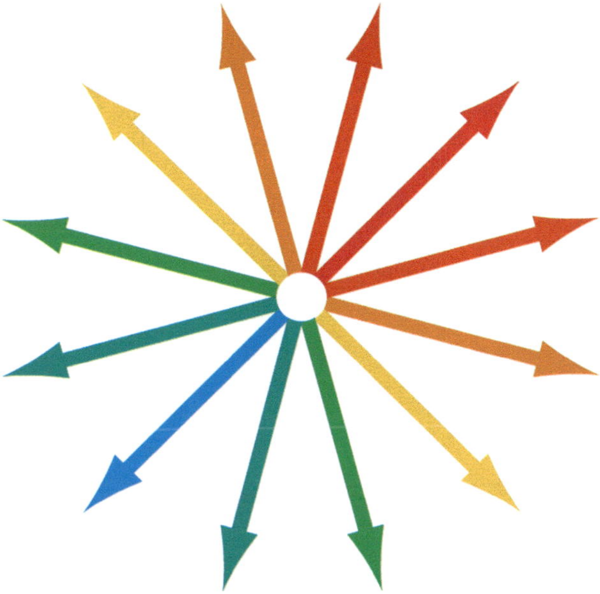

Fig. 20.5 Needle moving direction at supermicrosurgery

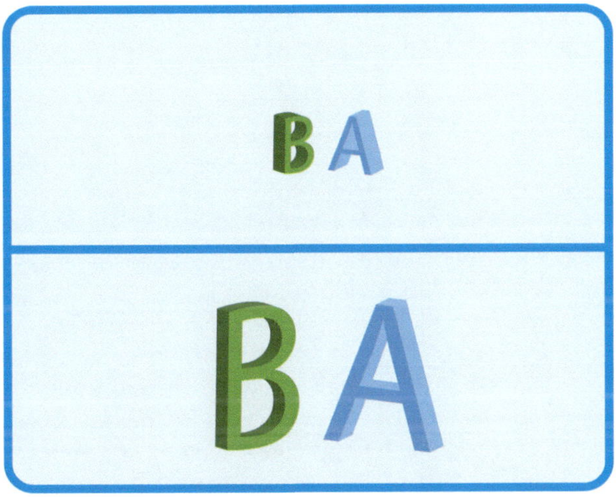

Fig. 20.6 The image of multiple view

References

1. Daniel RK, Taylor GI (1973) Distant transfer of an island flap by microvascular anastomoses. A clinical technique. Plast Reconstr Surg 52:111–117
2. Harii K, Omori S (1973) Use of the gastroepiploic vessels as recipient or donor vessels in the free transfer of composite flaps by microvascular anastomoses. Plast Reconstr Surg 52:541–548
3. Katz RD, Rosson GD, Taylor JA et al (2005) Robotics in microsurgery: use of a surgical robot to perform a free flap in a pig. Microsurgery 25:566–569

4. Koshima I, Inagawa K, Urushibara K et al (2000) Supermicrosurgical lymphaticovenular anastomosis for the treatment of lymphedema in the upper extremities. J Reconstr Microsurg 16:437–442
5. Koshima I, Inagawa K, Yamamoto M et al (2000) New microsurgical breast reconstruction using free paraumbilical perforator adiposal flaps. Plast Reconstr Surg 106:61–65
6. Koshima I, Soeda S, Yamasaki M et al (1988) The free or pedicled anteromedial thigh flap. Ann Plast Surg 21:480–485

21 Network

Catherine Jane Mohr

21.1 Introduction

Robotics affords a unique opportunity in surgery for introducing and seamlessly integrating new technologies to support and enhance both clinical decision making and the technical execution of surgical tasks. As distinct from traditional open or even minimally invasive surgical techniques such as laparoscopy or endoscopy, robotic surgery digitizes both the surgeon's vision and motion. Enormously complex technology is required to make this interposition of machinery between the surgeon's eyes and the patients' tissue, and the surgeon's hands and the surgical instruments, seamless and transparent to the surgeon (the "intuitive" of Intuitive Surgical™). Once a high-quality "intuitive" robotic platform has been developed, all the vision and motion that the surgeon experiences passes through an entirely digital step. The digitization provides an opportunity to expand the utility of the platform by injecting and integrating digital signals from other sources, or modifying the main signal stream to provide greater clinical value to the surgeon.

For a technologically unaided surgeon to be operating directly on a patient through an open incision, there are many conditions, constraints, and limitations that are so natural a part of surgical practice that we take them for granted:

1. Limitation of human vision – the surgeon's view of the patient's tissue is limited to reflected light in a spectrum visible to the human eye.
2. The condition of proximity – the patient must be within arm's reach of the surgeon and any assistants.
3. The constraint of scale – surgical tasks must be limited to a scale that is manipulable by the human hand (which has an average instrument manipulation accuracy of 220 μm) [5].

C.J. Mohr, M.D.
Department of Medical Research, Intuitive Surgical,
1266 Kifer Rd, Building 102, Sunnyvale 94086, CA, USA

Stanford School of Medicine, Palo Alto, CA, USA
e-mail: catherine.mohr@intusurg.com

P. Liverneaux et al. (eds.), *Telemicrosurgery*,
DOI 10.1007/978-2-8178-0391-3_21, © Springer-Verlag France 2013

4. The limitation of human proprioception – the surgeon must use his or her own visual and tactile observation of anatomy and proprioception to control where he or she places sutures or cuts.
5. The constraint of reality – the patient must actually exist.

Because of the digitization of the connection between the patient and surgeon, these conditions and constraints and limitations no longer apply when performing robotic surgery. In this chapter, we will examine the potential clinical benefit to be found in removing each of these constraints from the practice of surgery.

21.2 Removing the Limitations on Human Vision

Our unaided eyes are sensitive to only the visible spectrum (by definition), and even within the visible spectrum, not all the available information is captured by our eye. The primary limitation within the visible spectrum is that we discard spectral information. Light has no intrinsic color; we have rods and cones – sensors that are stimulated by certain wavelengths, or combination of wavelengths – and our brain performs quite a bit of complicated processing to perceive that as color; color is a "pigment of your imagination." We perceive 580 nm as yellow, but we also see red plus green (520+650 nm) as yellow which is why three-color displays are capable of reproducing a wide range of colors. Without the eye and the brain, there is no "yellow." There is a difference in the spectrum of these yellows, and in some cases a clinical significance to that difference, but our eyes perceive it as the same. In addition, our perception of color is extremely dependent on the color context, so a color may look radically different depending on what color it is in close proximity to (Fig. 21.1). Unlike the eye, however, cameras can be made that are sensitive to spectral differences, and a camera's capture of color is unaffected by the color environment surrounding that color. Cameras do, in general, have much lower dynamic range than our eyes, but they can make distinctions in the visible spectrum that our eyes can't.

Outside of the visible spectrum, wavelengths in the near infrared (NIR) have considerably greater penetration through tissue than any visible wavelengths, and we can use these wavelengths of light to help see what is below the surface. If we tag cancer, blood vessels, nerves, lymphatic structures, or other tissue types of interest with a dye that is fluorescent in the NIR, and use an NIR camera and light source, these structures become visible further below the surface than could be seen with visible spectrum lighting.

Spectral information and near-infrared fluorescence may be translated into a false color in the visible spectrum. The displayed reflected white light image may then be modified to incorporate this additional information and display these differences to the surgeon (Fig. 21.2).

A significant additional advantage of a completely digitized image is that it may be sent to more observers than the primary surgeon, including those at a distance. This facilitates collaboration and allows telementorship in which a surgeon at a distance may not only observe but also advise the operating surgeon by either verbal

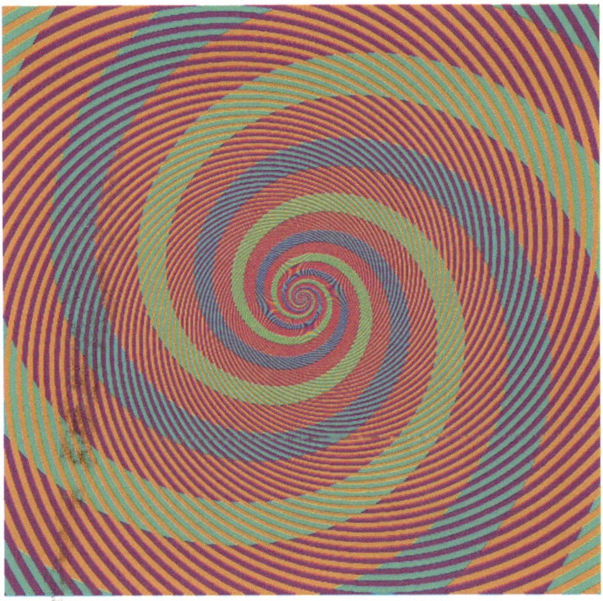

Fig. 21.1 Color illusion in which the *blue* and *green* spirals appear to be different colors because of the overlying colors (*fuchsia* and *orange* respectively) but are actually the same color (Image copyright A. Kitaoka 2003, used with permission of the author)

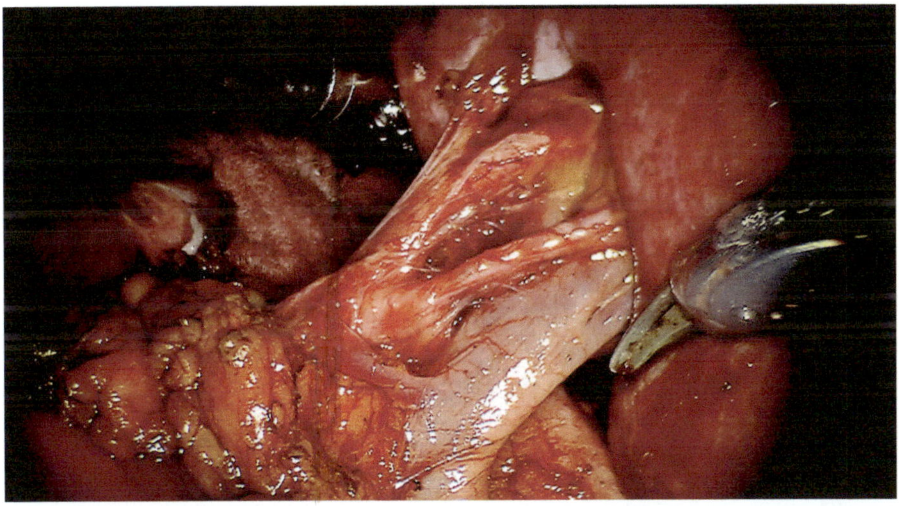

Fig. 21.2 Reflected white light image (**a**) and false color image (**b**) of renal arteries with indocyanine green IV injection and NIR fluorescence (Image copyright G. Wu, 2010, used with permission of the author)

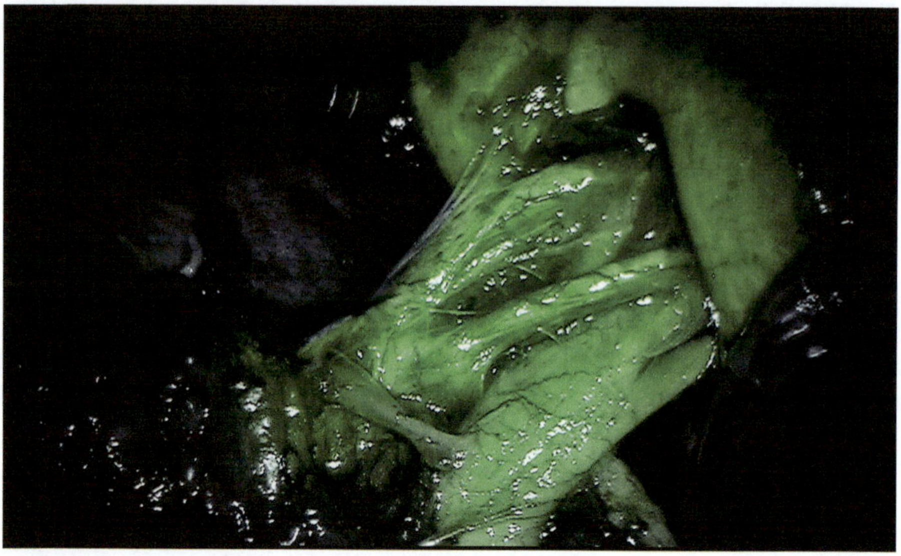

Fig. 21.2 (continued)

commands or by illustrating directly on the operative image for display to the operating surgeon in the surgeon console (Fig. 21.3).

21.3 Removing the Condition of Proximity

As the digitization of the image allowed sending it over a distance, fully digitizing the surgeon's hand motion by capturing the surgeon's input from the master controllers and turning this into a data stream for execution at the operational end of the robot allows the surgeon to move away from the "arm's length" constraint. In current practice with the da Vinci® surgical robot, the surgeon remains in the room operating from a console that is within 10 m of the patient. However, many have suggested benefits of allowing surgeons at a distance to operate on patients [4]. Studies were performed in Canada using the Zeus® system [1] and studies were performed with the ISI da Vinci® system under a grant by TATRC (Telemedicine and Advanced Technology Research Center) [7]. A setup similar to that shown in Fig. 21.4 would be required to perform surgery at a distance with the da Vinci system. There is no physical limit as to the distance over which control and video signals can be sent. Practical limitations such as available bandwidth and the effects of data transmission speed and reliability on motion quality, however, make operation at a distance of questionable value with present technology. The peak data transfer rates between the surgeon console and the da Vinci® patient side cart for the manipulation alone would overwhelm a majority of today's locally available Internet communications. In addition, delays imposed by variable communication latency and

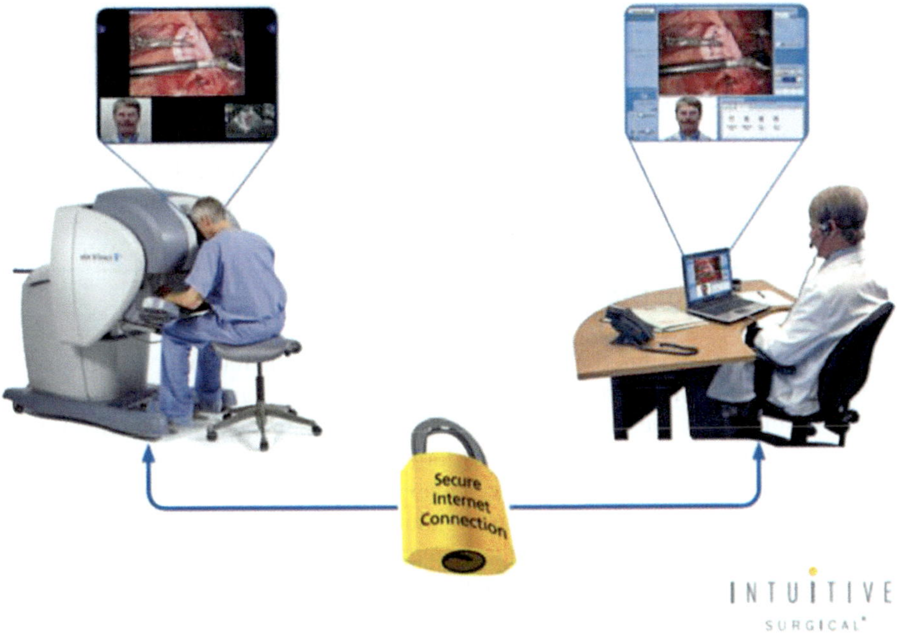

Fig. 21.3 Configuration for Intuitive Surgical's "Connect™" teleproctoring system which is used to allow experienced surgeons to remotely proctor new users of the da Vinci® system during their early cases

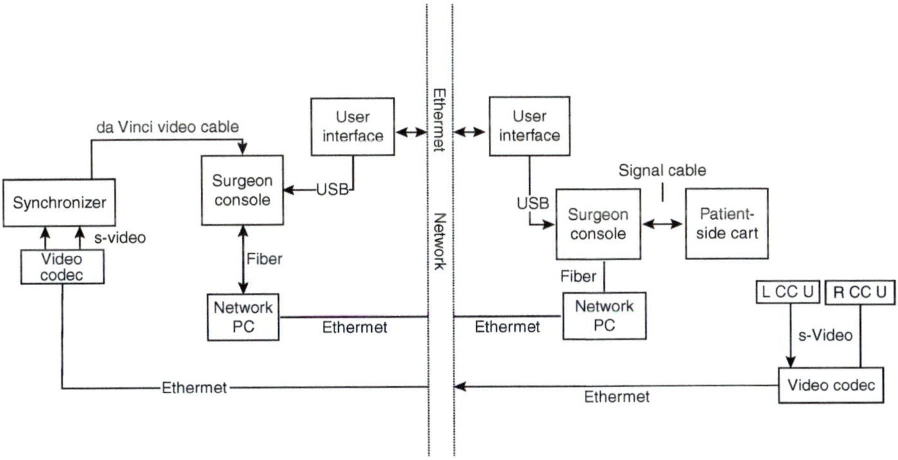

Fig. 21.4 Example of a setup for telesurgery with a stand-alone surgeon console operating the da Vinci® remotely

the fundamental upper limit of speed of light transmission of information means that manipulation tasks at a distance over a network would be subject to erratic performance, especially when delays become longer than 200 ms. Noise and delays for visual signals have been found to have much less of an effect on performance of surgical tasks over networks than manual delays [2], so telementoring and remote proctoring and collaboration will likely be used clinically for a long time before teleoperation becomes clinically viable outside of the study environment.

21.4 Removing the Constraint of Scale

In current robotic technology, physiologic tremor is filtered out, and the scale between the surgeon's hand and the motion being made can be made to be optimized for the size of the structures being operated upon. In the case of microsurgery, this is of particular interest, as allowing larger motions of the surgeons hand to be scaled very small will increase the precision with which surgical repair can be made and eliminate the effects of heartbeat, breathing, and physiologic tremor on instrument handling. With current robotic instrument technology, however, there are limitations to scales at which intuitive motion can still be preserved (currently about 7:1), as the hysteresis and friction in the instruments themselves start to produce unexpected motion for small motions at more extreme scales. These issues have the potential to be reduced by the development of specialized low-backlash instruments for microsurgery, but at present, these are not available. However, as previously discussed in the clinical sections, the currently available scaling factors already available with the da Vinci® do greatly increase surgeon comfort and performance with the added feature of tremor reduction.

21.5 Removing the Limit of Human Proprioception

The surgeon is highly trained in precise hand-eye coordination. A large part of surgical skill is the ability to place a needle or instrument tip at a precise position and orientation identified by the surgeon's eye. This highly accurate movement is possible because of constant visual feedback and the ability of the surgeon to correct his or her instrument trajectory with a combination of visual and proprioceptive feedback. Surgeons using robotics are capable of achieving similar or better relative accuracies, but in addition, because of position measurements on the joints of the robot, an advantage robotics provides is the ability to calculate the absolute measurement of position of the tip of an instrument rather than simply the relative position. This allows additional data such as "no fly" zones or navigation or constraints on motion of the tip to be imposed to either protect structures, prevent dissection or drilling below a certain level, or to provide a "stencil" for an instrument to follow a prescribed contour. While the current da Vinci® system does not provide these features, they are possible to implement in a robotic system where tip positions are calculable from measured joint angles.

21.6 Removing the Constraint of Reality

Surgical training has traditionally been achieved with practice on real patients. Full digitization of motion and vision means that an entirely synthetic representation of the patient's tissues may be presented to the surgeon at the console with no change in the nature of the physical interactions that the surgeon has with the console. Simulation allows surgical skills to be practiced without the morbidity of patients being learned upon, and the same exercise may be presented until mastery is achieved. A study in 2002 showed surgical residents trained to perform laparoscopic surgery using simulation with virtual reality simulators were more proficient and made fewer errors in the operating room than those who received no virtual reality simulated education [6], and initial studies with robotic simulators have supported the validity of currently available simulators [3]. In addition, because the entire motion of the surgeon's hands is captured in the execution of the task, quality metrics such as accuracy, economy, or quality of motion may be employed to evaluate the surgeons' performance and measure progress in mastery.

Conclusion

The opportunities for bringing in new technologies to support and enhance clinical outcomes are not limited to the items discussed here, but as more technologies are developed, the robotic platforms of the future will allow integration of these new technologies to support and enhance clinical abilities for the surgeon, ultimately for the benefit of the patients.

References

1. Anvari M, McKinley C, Stein H (2005) Establishment of the world's first telerobotic remote surgical service: for provision of advanced laparoscopic surgery in a rural community. Ann Surg 241:460–464
2. Hanly EJ, Miller BE, Kumar R et al (2006) Mentoring console improves collaboration and teaching in surgical robotics. J Laparoendosc Adv Surg Tech A 16:445–451
3. Kenney PA, Wszolek MF, Gould JJ et al (2009) Face, content, and construct validity of dV-trainer, a novel virtual reality simulator for robotic surgery. Urology 73:1288–1292
4. Marescaux J, Leroy J, Rubino F et al (2002) Transcontinental robot-assisted remote telesurgery: feasibility and potential applications. Ann Surg 235:487–492
5. Runge A, Hofer M, Dittrich E et al (2011) Manual accuracy in comparison with a miniature master slave device – preclinical evaluation for ear surgery. Stud Health Technol Inform 163:524–530
6. Seymour NE, Gallagher AG, Roman SA et al (2002) Virtual reality training improves operating room performance: results of a randomized, double-blinded study. Ann Surg 236:458–463; discussion 463–464
7. TATRC Report No. 04-03 (2004) Integrated research team final report: surgical robotics – the next steps

Postface

Seen from afar, and, given my incompetence in the subject, from far afar, the topic of this book, telemicrosurgery is quite exemplary. Exemplary by its merging of knowledge drawn from diverse areas of science, exemplary by its combination of basic insight and of technical expertise, exemplary also by the intimate link between the performance of the actors/operators and the benefit to the spectators/patients. Bringing together the most recent advances in widely spread fields, always at the forefront of progress and drawing on seemingly unrelated areas, telemicrosurgery achieves triple precision in space, in size and in action. It is a celebration of science, technology and ingenuity that is changing life.

We must be deeply thankful to all those who have contributed to the saga of telemicrosurgery, to its emergence, its development, its experimental assessment, and of course foremost to its introduction into clinical practice for the great benefit of patients. The present volume aptly describes the activities in the field. It takes stock and paints the panorama as seen by major contributors, those who hold the cards in their hand, qui tiennent les cartes en Main!

Jean Marie Lehn Ph.D.
Nobel Prize in Chemistry 1987
ISIS, Université de Strasbourg, 8 allée Gaspard Monge
F-67000, Strasbourg, France
e-mail:lehn@unistra.fr

P. Liverneaux et al. (eds.), *Telemicrosurgery*,
DOI 10.1007/978-2-8178-0391-3, © Springer-Verlag France 2013

GPSR Compliance

The European Union's (EU) General Product Safety Regulation (GPSR) is a set of rules that requires consumer products to be safe and our obligations to ensure this.

If you have any concerns about our products, you can contact us on ProductSafety@springernature.com

In case Publisher is established outside the EU, the EU authorized representative is:

Springer Nature Customer Service Center GmbH
Europaplatz 3
69115 Heidelberg, Germany

Batch number: 10732566

Printed by Printforce, the Netherlands